BROILER CHICKENS: WELFARE IN PRACTICE

BROILER CHICKENS: WELFARE IN PRACTICE

Andy Butterworth, Ingrid de Jong, Joy Mench, Lotta Berg, and Mohan Raj

Series Editor: Xavier Manteca Vilanova

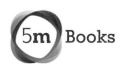 Books

Published by
5m Books Ltd
Lings, Great Easton
Essex CM6 2HH, UK
www.5mbooks.com

A Catalogue record for this book is available from the British Library

ISBN 9781789180152

Book layout by KSPM, 8 Wood Road, Codsall, Wolverhampton, WV8 1DB
Printed by Hobbs The Printers Ltd, Totton, Hampshire

Photos by the authors unless otherwise indicated

Contents

3   Influences of housing and management on broiler welfare

4   Health and disease impacts on broiler welfare

Contributors

Andy Butterworth (andy.butterworth@icloud.com)

Andy was a practitioner in mixed veterinary practice in the UK, and a veterinary researcher at the University of Bristol Vet School. Andy works on animal health, animal welfare, disease and production systems, and consults in the area of practical animal welfare improvement. He helps to write national and international animal welfare standards and is part of the international training businesses AWT (www.awtraining.com) and WelfareMax (www.welfaremax.com). Andy has been a member of the EFSA Animal Health and Welfare Panel, and is a current member of the Council of Management of the *British Poultry Science Journal*, and of the UK Defra Animal Welfare Committee, which advises UK Government on Animal Health and Welfare. He has over 300 books, patents, and scientific and trade publications, and has spoken at conferences and provided training and consultancy in many parts of the world.

Ingrid de Jong (ingrid.dejong@wur.nl)

Ingrid de Jong studied Animal Sciences at Wageningen University, with a focus on ethology, animal physiology and immunology and obtained her doctorate in animal physiology at the University of Groningen, the Netherlands. She is working as a senior scientific researcher at Wageningen Livestock Research, Wageningen University & Research, where she coordinates research projects related to welfare of broilers, broiler breeders and laying hens for the EU, national government and private companies. She has published 55 scientific papers, in addition to various book chapters, conference papers and reports, and has been invited speaker at various international conferences on animal welfare.

Joy Mench (jamench@ucdavis.edu)

Joy Mench is a professor emeritus at the University of California, Davis (UCD). She received her doctorate in Ethology at the University of Sussex in the UK, carried out postdoctoral research at Cornell University, and was a professor at the University of Maryland, College Park, for 10 years before moving to UCD in 1995. Her area of emphasis is the behaviour and welfare of captive and managed animals, with a particular focus on poultry. She has published hundreds of papers, book chapters and books on these topics. At UCD, she taught classes on animal welfare, animal ethics, and professional ethics. She consults extensively on animal welfare for a range of stakeholders, including retailers, farmers, trade groups, government agencies, and animal welfare organizations. She was recently named a Fellow of the Poultry Science Association and the International Society for Applied Ethology.

Lotta Berg (lotta.berg@slu.se)

Lotta (Charlotte) Berg is a professor in Animal Environment and Health at the Swedish University of Agricultural Sciences, and started her research career at the same university where she received a doctorate based on a thesis focusing on the epidemiology and prevention of management-related diseases of welfare relevance in broilers. She has since been working mainly with poultry and other farm animals, but also with other species. She is interested in the interface between wildlife and farmed animals, including welfare and zoonotic disease aspects (One Health). She has worked for the Swedish government, writing and updating animal welfare legislation nationally and internationally and supporting the operational control authorities in their animal welfare work. She holds a Diplomate Certificate of the European

College of Animal Welfare and Behavioural Medicine; subspeciality of Welfare Science, Ethics and Law. She has been a member of the Animal Health and Animal Welfare (AHAW) panel at the European Food Safety Authority (EFSA), Parma and is currently the Swedish National Contact Point with reference to animal welfare issues at slaughter and on-farm killing.

Mohan Raj (abmraj1957@gmail.com)

Mohan Raj is a veterinary scientist specialised in farm animal welfare, especially during stunning and slaughter for human consumption and killing during disease outbreaks. He has published over 100 papers as international scientific journal articles, book chapters, reviews and conference papers and has been an invited speaker at international conferences on animal welfare. He served as a member of the Animal Health and Welfare Penal of the European Food Safety Authority (EFSA). He is also a member of the Council of Management of the *British Poultry Science Journal*.

Xavier Manteca (xavier.manteca@uab.es)

Xavier Manteca Vilanova received his BVSc and doctorate from the Autonomous University of Barcelona and an MSc in Applied Animal Behaviour and Animal Welfare from the University of Edinburgh. Currently, he is professor of animal behaviour and animal welfare at the School of Veterinary Science in Barcelona. He has published extensively and is diplomate of the European College of Animal Welfare and Behavioural Medicine.

Foreword

Animal welfare is an essential element of modern animal production and is grounded on ethical concerns that derive from the fact that animals are sentient beings, i.e. able to suffer and experience emotions. Moreover, improving animal welfare may have additional benefits. As many welfare problems have a detrimental effect on production, improving the welfare of farm animals often has positive effects on their production performance. Also, improving animal welfare may contribute to human health by reducing the risk of zoonotic diseases as well as the use of antimicrobials.

Broiler chickens are by far the most numerous of all terrestrial farm animals. It has been estimated that roughly 70 billion broilers are slaughtered every year in the world and this number is expected to increase over the next few years, mainly in developing countries. Therefore, and based on the number of animals affected, welfare problems of broilers must be ranked among the most important of all farm animal welfare problems.

Broiler welfare is a very active area of research and there is a vast amount of information in scientific journals and technical reports. The objective of this book is to provide a succinct, easy-to-read summary of the available literature on broiler welfare. The book follows a practical approach and is addressed mainly to field veterinarians, animal welfare advisors and farmers.

The book includes seven chapters. The first three chapters describe the main welfare problems of broilers (Chapters 1 and 2) and broiler breeders (Chapter 3). Chapter 4 is devoted to an area that, despite its relevance, is frequently overlooked in many books on animal welfare, namely the welfare of chicks at the hatchery. Chapter 5 discusses welfare assessment methods for broilers and Chapter 6 addresses the welfare implications of on-farm and casualty slaughter of broilers. Finally, Chapter 7 builds on all previous chapters and provides a very useful summary of practical strategies to improve broiler welfare.

The book has been written by an international team of well-known, highly respected animal welfare scientists led by Dr Andy Butterworth. All of them have both an impressive track record of scientific publications in animal welfare as well as a vast amount of practical experience in broiler welfare.

I really hope that this book will be very useful to all those involved in broiler production and will contribute to improve the welfare of chickens.

Prof. Xavier Manteca

Series Editor

Farm Animal Welfare Education Centre (FAWEC)

School of Veterinary Science

Universitat Autònoma de Barcelona, Spain

Introduction

Animal welfare has become in many countries an integral part of animal husbandry. Whereas in some parts of the world animal welfare is considered because of moral concern, for cultural reasons or its link to productivity, in other parts, it has mainly been enforced by legislation, encouraged through assurance schemes or demanded by retailers. The latter set of drivers has put pressure on many producers worldwide as they need to adjust their systems to proscribed requirements. This initially may seem to disadvantage their market position compared to countries where animal welfare is not as much part of the political agenda or societal debate. Animal welfare is, however, much more than just the guidelines set by policymakers. In fact, improving animal welfare can be very favourable for productivity when integrated well in farm management. As most animal welfare issues are multifactorial, such as broiler lameness, case-to-case solutions may be needed.

This book is part of a series of short, practical books on the welfare of farmed animals. The series covers what is currently known about the welfare requirements of specific animal species and how to put this into practice. Its aim is to provide people in different countries with a tool to improve animal welfare through scientifically based information presented in a concise, easy to understand way. *Broiler Chickens: Welfare in Practice* focuses on chickens kept commercially. The book is aimed at farmers, stockworkers and animal handlers, and additionally as a reference for smallholders, animal scientists and agricultural students.

The chapters in this book are written by esteemed researchers. They have studied chicken behaviour, welfare and production for many years and, besides their roles as scientists, they actively engage in knowledge exchange by advising farmers and other stakeholders.

- **Chapter 1** Broiler breeder welfare – considers the welfare issues relating to the parent birds who produce the eggs that will become the final stage broilers.
- **Chapter 2** Hatchery welfare – looks at the multiple factors that influence the health and welfare of the chick as it hatches in the commercial hatchery.
- **Chapter 3** Influences of housing and management on the welfare of production broilers – considers the management, housing and farm environment factors which so greatly influence the welfare of broilers during their short production lives.
- **Chapter 4** Health and disease impacts on broiler welfare – how can we protect the health of broiler chickens, and when disease occurs, how can we monitor and reduce its impacts?
- **Chapter 5** On-farm and casualty slaughter welfare of broilers – how to deal with sick and injured broiler chickens on-farm.
- **Chapter 6** Welfare assessment methods for broiler chickens – methods to assess (and hence to improve) broiler welfare.
- **Chapter 7** What can we do to improve animal welfare – how we can use science, management, biosecurity, veterinary input and animal based measures to improve the welfare of the billions of broilers farmed each year across the world.

The suggestions given in this book are based on scientific studies. This is, however, no guarantee that a certain strategy will be effective on every farm, in every situation. Please be cautious with making changes in the management and monitor the animals closely, and consult with the veterinarian if required.

CHAPTER 1

Broiler breeder welfare

INGRID DE JONG AND ANDY BUTTERWORTH

Broiler breeding is the process of genetic selection for desirable characteristics of the final product: the broiler chicken. Desirable characteristics include those related to both technical performance, such as, food conversion ratio and growth profile, but also to health and welfare, such as, mortality and leg health. For the female breeders, that is, the hens producing the eggs that will become a broiler chicken, reproductive characteristics, such as, the number of hatching eggs produced is an important selection criterion. Figure 1.1 shows the breeding pyramid. The structure of the pyramid shows that a relatively small number of birds are present at the top of the pyramid – the purebred lines – and that successive cycles of production lead to a large number of chickens at the bottom of the pyramid (the broilers, the final generation). As an example, annually about 7500 million broilers are reared in the European Union (EU), produced by approximately 60 million broiler breeders (Hiemstra and Ten Napel, 2011). Broilers are always crosses of at least three or four genetic lines.

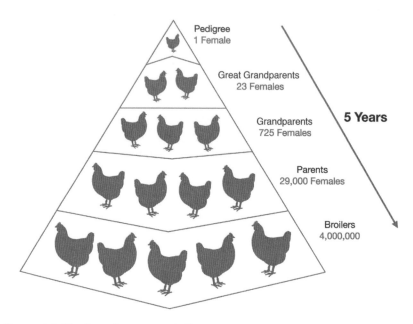

Figure 1.1 The breeding pyramid. The pedigree lines at the top of the pyramid are the first step in the production of broiler chickens, shown at the bottom of the pyramid. These are usually the result of the crossing of three to four genetic lines. One female at the top has a genetic influence on approximately 4 million broiler chickens at the bottom of the pyramid. It takes 4 to 5 years for a change in characteristics at the top to be represented in the progeny at the bottom.

Three large breeding companies dominate the market for broiler chickens worldwide: Aviagen, Cobb-Vantress, and Hubbard. Each breeding company has its own pure genetic lines, known as the pedigree stock (see Figure 1.1). The pedigree stock are housed at geographically spread out breeding sites that are used for genetic selection, and which meet high biosecurity requirements. In addition, relatives of the pedigree stock are housed in commercial environments to test their performance under the conditions in which the birds are housed in practice. Great grandparents and grandparents are produced at multiplication sites that are controlled by the breeding companies. The three different breeding companies all have different parent stock (broiler breeder) lines, targeted at different market requirements worldwide (Hiemstra and Ten Napel, 2011). This chapter focuses on the welfare of broiler breeders, that is, the male and female chickens that produce the eggs that become broiler chickens.

Housing and management of broiler breeders

Here we summarise the more detailed information on housing and management which can be found in EFSA (2010), de Jong and Swalander (2012) and de Jong and van Emous (2017). Biosecurity levels are usually high in both rearing and production environments, as the health of the breeders may potentially affect the health of a large number of broiler chickens.

Rearing

Broiler breeder males and females are usually reared on separate farms and transported to the production farm at between 18 and 22 weeks of age. The aim of the rearing period is to produce chickens with the ideal weight, body weight uniformity and sexual stage of maturity when they enter the production farm. Group sizes within each house differ between countries and farms, but usually female groups consist of several thousand birds and rearing farms can have more than one house on the same location. As a lower number of males are needed to produce the fertilised eggs (see below), group sizes of males are much smaller than groups of females. Broiler breeders are usually housed on a floor covered with substrate, such as wood shavings, peat moss or straw. Both windowed houses and houses without windows are used, dependent on local traditions or regulations. In some countries, depending on the climate, open-sided houses are used, in which one side of the house is covered with wire mesh and raisable curtains. The manure becomes an integrated part of the litter. Breeding companies advise the producer to provide perches or raised platforms to train the birds to jump up onto the raised slatted floor in the production phase (see below). Water is provided through cups, nipples or bell drinkers, and is sometimes provided on the raised slats from about 6 weeks of age onwards to train the birds to use the slats. Feed can be provided as mash, crumb or pellet, and is usually provided in the litter area in feeding pans or via chain feeders. Some farms use spin feeders, which distribute the feed in the litter to promote foraging behaviour, and this may improve skeletal growth and mobility. Only pellet feed can be used in spin feeders. Providing sufficient feeder space during rearing is essential to prevent aggression around feeding time and the resulting injuries arising from competition for feed. Figure 1.2 shows a few examples of rearing houses.

With respect to stocking density and lighting, guidelines produced by the breeding companies are usually applied. Common densities are 4–8 males or 7–10 females/m² with lower stocking densities in open-sided houses.

A lighting programme of 8 hours light and 16 hours darkness is usually used during rearing. Light intensity may vary, for example, due to the presence of windows, but as a guideline 20 lux at animal height may be used in non-windowed houses. When injurious pecking behaviour occurs, farmers often reduce the light intensity. The feeding regime is strictly controlled, which means that breeder birds are fed according to the desired growth profile.

During early growth, birds usually receive an unrestricted (*ad libitum*) amount of feed. Thereafter, they will receive their feed in controlled daily portions to prevent them from growing faster than the desired growth curve and to grow at a rate to reach their target weight and stage of development at the start of production. Although in many countries breeders are fed at least once daily, so-called 'skip-a-day' feeding programmes are also used. There are different types of skip-a-day feeding programmes, such as 6/1 (six days feeding and one day without feed), 5/2 (five feeding days within a week and two days without feed) or 4/3

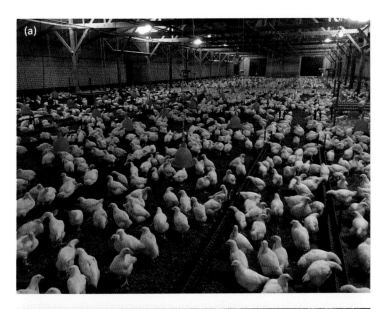

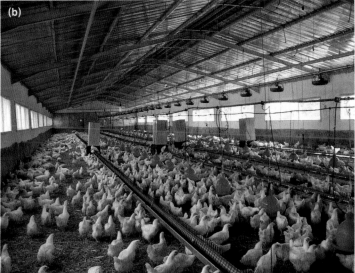

Figure 1.2 Example of rearing houses: (a) indoor housing without windows (provided by Rick van Emous, Wageningen University and Research); (b) open-sided rearing house in Africa (provided by Hubbard).

(four feeding days a week and three days without feed). With these skip-a-day feeding programmes, the daily feed amount is higher on feeding days. These programmes may result in better body weight uniformity due to 'less severe' competition around feeding.

The welfare consequences of the various feeding programmes are discussed below. Water can be provided unrestricted, but many farms apply a restricted water regime to reduce the risk of wet litter. Water can be provided during a restricted period of the day, or on a fixed water : feed ratio, or the water pressure can be lowered so that the birds have to drink for longer to gain the same amount of liquid. During the rearing period broiler breeders receive several vaccinations to protect against common poultry diseases. Culling is done to remove birds that are the wrong sex for the rearing group (sexing errors), are sick or remain small (runts).

The broiler breeder flocks that produce slower-growing broiler chickens (for example, for organic or free-range broiler production) usually have different feeding regimes than those described above. These breeder flocks are genetically predisposed to grow more slowly than breeders of the so-called fast-growing broiler strains. This means that either one sex (usually the female) or both sexes receive a much less controlled feeding regimen during the rearing period to reach their target weight at the start of production. Water restriction is also not used for these flocks, or to a much lesser extent.

Production period

The production period usually starts around 18 to 22 weeks of age and lasts until 60 to 65 weeks of age. The main goal of the production period is to produce a high number of fertilised eggs of good uniformity and quality. In the majority of the breeder flocks worldwide natural mating is used, although in some countries cage systems with artificial insemination are used. Here we will focus on systems with natural mating.

Males and females are transported from the production farm to the rearing farm. Group sizes on the rearing farm vary, but houses usually contain several thousand birds and several similar sized houses can be often be present on one farm. During production, broiler breeders are housed in systems with a partially littered floor, and a raised slatted floor area, on which the nests and usually also the drinkers are placed. The ratio littered : slatted floor varies, but most commonly is two-thirds litter area and one-third raised slatted floor. Sometimes perches are provided on the slatted area, or in the litter area.

Colony cages for broiler breeders do exist, although they are not very commonly used. These contain nests, perches, and a scratching area and a slatted floor. Feed can be provided in feeder chains or pans. Males and females have separate feeding systems, which allow feed to be controlled separately for males and females, with the general intention to control body weight, particularly in the male. Male feeding systems are usually higher so that females are unable to reach them. In female systems so-called 'grills' are placed on the feeders so that males cannot put their heads in them (males are larger and their heads are wider). Water can be provided in bell drinkers, cups or nipples. Some farmers supply additional grains or shells in the litter in the afternoon, and on some farms enrichments such as pecking stones or lucerne bales are provided in the litter area. Figure 1.3 shows some examples of production houses.

Dependent on region and climate, indoor houses with or without windows or curtained houses are used. Artificial lighting is used in addition to natural light to stimulate reproduction. To promote the sexual development of the birds, the duration of the light period is gradually increased after arrival of the chickens on the breeder farm. The production period usually lasts until the birds reach 60–65 weeks of age, and the parent stock of slower-growing broiler strains usually have a longer production period than parent stock of fast-growing broilers.

The stocking density during the production period varies between 5–7.5 birds/m^2. Males are introduced into the flock at the start of the

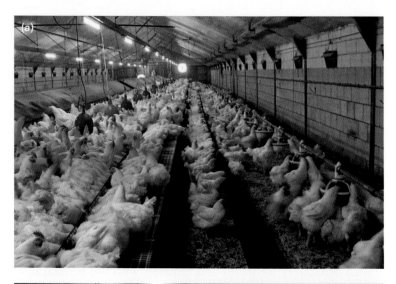

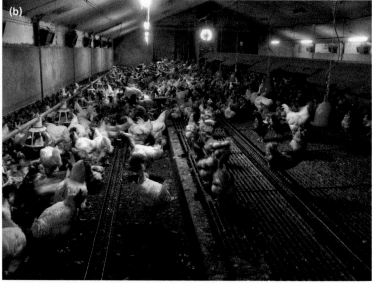

Figure 1.3 Examples of production houses: (a) indoor house with parent stock of fast-growing broiler strains (photo: Rick van Emous, Wageningen University & Research); (b) indoor house with parent stock of a slower-growing broiler strain, that is, dwarf females and a conventional male.

production period. At this time the males make up 8–11% of the flock. The number of males decreases to 6–9% at the end of the production period due to selection (removal of poor performing birds), culling and mortality. 'Spiking' is a common practice in broiler breeder farming, and takes place when a proportion of the existing mature males (inactive or poor performing males) are replaced by younger males to maintain the production of fertile eggs. However, this practice of introducing young male breeders into the existing flock involves the risk of introduction of disease, and spiking may also lead to aggression between males. For parent stock of standard fast-growing broilers, feed is also provided in restricted quantities during the production period, but to a much lesser extent as compared to the rearing period, especially after the peak of production (>30 weeks of age).

Welfare issues

Beak and toe trimming

Beak and toe trimming procedures are common in broiler breeder flocks, although in some countries they are (partially) prohibited by law (de Jong and van Emous, 2017). Both male and female broiler breeders may be beak trimmed. This can be done in the hatchery, by the infrared 'beak tipping' or 'beak treatment' method, or on the farm at a few days of age by hot-blade beak trimming. For females, beak trimming is used to prevent feather damage and injuries due to feather pecking and cannibalistic pecking. For males, beak trimming is usually used to prevent damage to the females due to the mating behaviour of the males. In countries where females are not allowed to be beak trimmed, such as the UK, Poland, Sweden, and recently in the Netherlands, in actuality, only low numbers of problems related to injurious pecking are reported in flocks with breeders of fast-growing broiler chicken strains. For breeder flocks of slower-growing strains, there is little experience with keeping flocks with intact beaks. As an example, in the Netherlands there is now a ban on beak trimming for female breeders of fast-growing strains, and a postponed ban for breeder flocks of slower-growing strains. There are only a few countries globally in which males are not beak trimmed but this does not seem to have resulted in excessive levels of damage to the females. Figure 1.4 shows a non-beak trimmed and beak trimmed male breeder.

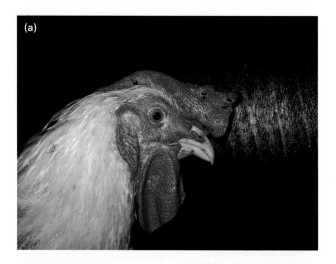

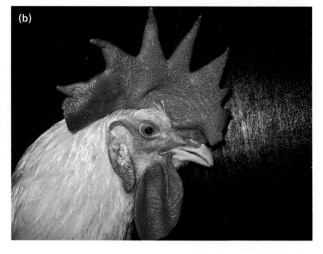

Figure 1.4
Male with
(a) intact beak;
(b) beak trimmed
by infrared
method in the
hatchery.

Pecking behaviour towards the feeder or other parts of the pen may smooth and blunt the sharp tip of the beak and promoting this smoothening may help to control damage caused by injurious pecking, when beaks are not trimmed. For example, rough surfaces can be installed in plastic feeders that smoothen the beaks in a natural way when feeding.

Apart from beak trimming, the inner toes of the males are treated in the hatchery (the toe is tipped so that there is no sharp nail), to prevent damage from this toe to the female during mating. In contrast to beak trimming, this procedure is used worldwide. The concern is that if toes are not trimmed it will result in severe damage (wounds at the thigh area) and increased mortality in the female breeders. In the Netherlands, a ban on toe clipping is foreseen in the next few years, and studies are in progress to determine whether or not a ban on toe clipping is likely to result in unacceptable levels of female injuries. Preliminary results showed that in a flock (parent stock of fast-growing broiler strains) with males with intact toes, increased female mortality due to injuries was found, while in another flock (parent stock of slower-growing strains) no effect on the females was found. However, this topic needs to be further studied in a larger sample of flocks. Another area for research is whether or not management measures could be introduced to reduce the risk of injuries in females when males are not toe clipped, as this subject has, until now, not been studied.

Restricted or 'controlled' feeding programmes

Parent stock of so-called fast-growing broiler strains have their feed restricted, especially during the rearing period, to prevent health issues related to high body weight, and associated reproduction problems when adult (EFSA, 2010). The very high feed intake and growth rate these birds can achieve when they are not feed restricted is related to the genetic selection for efficient growth of the final stage progeny – the broiler chickens. Unrestricted feeding results in low egg production, low egg quality and low persistency of lay. However, restricted feeding also leads to welfare problems, including hunger, altered behavioural patterns and frustration of the feeding motivation. This duality of effect is known as the 'broiler breeder paradox' (Decuypere et al., 2006).

The restricted feeding programme during the rearing period results in altered behaviours, some of which are indicative of hunger, and frustration of the feeding motivation. These behaviours include stereotypic object pecking (pecking at non-food items repetitively), pacing (stereotyped walking) and very high activity levels of the birds. In addition, physiological indicators of stress, such as, increased plasma corticosterone concentrations and increased heterophil : lymphocyte ratios in the blood have been reported to be associated with hunger. Although studies in the early 1990s reported that restricted feeding of broiler breeders had a negative effect on the welfare of the birds, so far, no real solution to this problem has been found. Various studies have focused on nutritional measures to alleviate the stress related to restricted feeding, for instance, by diluting the diet with fibrous material to promote feelings of satiety (Hocking et al., 2004; Sandilands et al., 2006; Nielsen et al., 2011). Examples of fibrous material that have been added to diets are oat hulls, cellulose, wheat bran, sugar beet pulp and cottonseed meal. Other studies have changed the energy : protein ratio in the diet (van Emous et al., 2015). Some of these 'modified' diets have been shown to reduce behaviours indicative of hunger and frustration, but none of the measures used so far have been able to completely prevent 'metabolic hunger' and so far these measures are not applied on a large scale in practice. Another possible solution that has been examined is the inclusion of a chemical appetite suppressant in the feed (calcium propionate). Studies showed that this could be effective in reducing behavioural indicators related to hunger and frustration (Sandilands et al., 2006), but there is ongoing discussion on the acceptability of such components as diet ingredients. These added ingredients may cause the birds to feel ill, and thus be a cause of welfare issues by themselves. Other measures to reduce the negative effects of restricted feeding, such as increasing the daily feeding frequency or distributing feed in the litter, have not proven to be effective thus far. Studies that compared the different feeding pro-grammes, that is, daily feeding versus various skip-a-day programmes, did not show benefits of any of these programmes with respect to broiler welfare (D'Eath et al., 2009; EFSA, 2010; de Jong and Guemene, 2011). It should be noted that the majority of studies have previously focused on females, and that little is known on the effect of restricted diets on male bird welfare. EFSA (2010) reported that males are relatively more restricted than females during the rearing period.

During the production period, the relative level of feed restriction is lower compared to the rearing period, especially after the peak of lay. Behavioural and physiological signs of hunger and frustration can be observed during production, especially in the early weeks, but to a much lesser extent when compared to the rearing period (EFSA, 2010).

Parent stock of so-called slower-growing broiler strains, where selec-tion pressure for efficient growth is much reduced compared to the conventional fast-growing strains, do not need to be feed restricted, or if so, to a much lesser extent. Any restriction required will depend on the breed and broiler chicken strain, and this will also influence whether both the male and females, or only the females, should be feed restricted. As an example, dwarf breeder females that do not need to be feed restricted can be mated with a regular, fast-growing male, and this male may need to be feed restricted. To produce broiler chickens that grow more slowly, these females can be mated with males with a genetic capacity for slow growth and in that case neither the males nor females need to be restricted (or to a much lesser extent). The use of parent stock of slower-growing broiler strains thus presents a potential commercial-scale solution to the problem of feed restriction, however, the majority of the broiler chickens produced worldwide are of the con-ventional, fast-growing strains. A change towards other genotypes of broiler chicken, and thus a change in the genetics of parent stock, will be dependent on market requirements, and so far only niche markets have changed towards the use of other genetic strains of broiler chickens (de Jong and Guemene, 2011).

Restricted water supply

Broiler breeders are quite frequently subjected to a restricted water supply. Restriction is generally applied to reduce water spillage related to excessive pecking at the drinker, which may result in wet litter, which is in turn a risk factor for footpad dermatitis and hock burn. There is little scientific evidence about the effects of restricted water supply on broiler breeder welfare, but it is generally considered that water restriction as a management practice has negative effects on broiler breeder welfare and should not be considered necessary. Breeding companies advise that broiler breeders be given continuous access to fresh and clean water (Aviagen, 2018).

Mating behaviour, injuries and feather cover

Male broiler breeders may show rough behaviour towards females when mating, resulting in damage to the feather cover and injuries (Millman et al., 2000; de Jong and Guemene, 2011). Pecking and chasing of females, and forced copulation, may result in females hiding from the males on the slatted area and in the nests. Further, the 'usual' repertoire of courtship behaviour that precedes mating in birds reared at low density, has hardly been observed in commercial broiler breeder flocks (de Jong et al., 2009). An important aspect of preventing aggression by males towards females at mating is to ensure that males do not reach sexual maturity at an earlier stage than females. But even if males are matched with respect to maturity with females, the males may still act aggressively towards females. It has been suggested that this problem can be alleviated by separating males from females during a part of the day, or even reducing the contact between males and females to once every 2 days. Male mating frequency in commercial houses is estimated to be five to ten times higher than under natural conditions, and this is thought to be one cause of the rough mating behaviour of the males towards females. The concept of separating males from females during a part of the day has been tested on a Dutch commercial farm and did not negatively affect performance results, but needs to be tested and developed further at commercial level (de Jong and van Emous, 2017). Another measure that may positively affect mating behaviour is the application of UV-enriched light, and this has resulted in changes in mating behaviour (Jones et al., 2001). Further, providing vertical cover panels in the litter area enables hens to hide from the males (Leone and Estevez, 2008).

Good feather cover may protect females from damage by males during mating, and improve thermoregulation. The feather cover of parent stock of fast-growing broiler strains shows a rapid decrease in quality with increasing age (Figure 1.5) and this is associated with a risk of skin damage and wounds (Figure 1.6). One reason for the deteriorating feather cover can be mating activity, but it is also thought that feed composition plays a role. Specific amino acids are important for feather

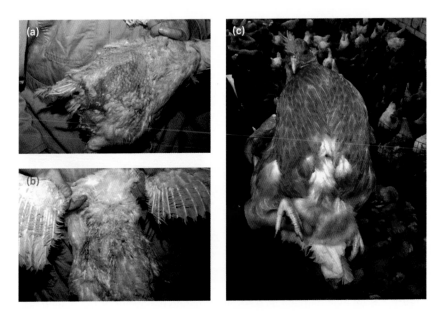

Figure 1.5 Examples of feather damage in broiler breeders: (a) and (b) severely damaged feathers; (c) slightly damaged feather cover.

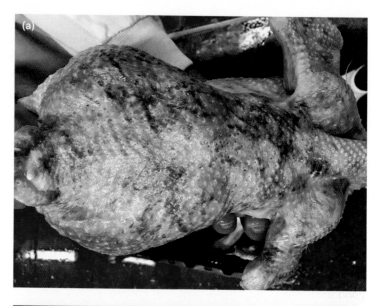

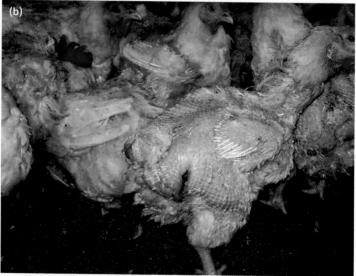

Figure 1.6 (a) Skin damage as a result of mating behaviour of the male (measured at slaughter after de-feathering); (b) a hen with a very poor feather cover at the end of the laying period, and a wound caused by mating.

development and a deficiency leads to a worsening in the quality of the feather cover. Furthermore, with reduced stocking density during rearing and production the quality of the feather cover improves (de Jong and van Emous, 2017). Competition around the feeders, for example, especially during the rearing period, may cause aggressive pecking or result in birds walking over each other, which can also damage the feather cover. Generally, the parent stock of fast-growing broiler strains has worse feather cover at the end of production than the parent stock of slower-growing broiler strains (Figure 1.6).

Environmental enrichment

Chickens prefer resting on an elevated structure, and this is also the case for broiler breeders. It has been shown that broiler breeders make good use of elevated perches and plastic perforated platforms for resting (Gebhardt-Henrich et al., 2017, 2018). During the rearing period, raised slatted areas are often offered to train the breeders to use vertical space because, during the production period, resources such as nests and water will (partially) be provided on raised slatted area. However, the amount of slatted area (proportion of the total area) provided during rearing is usually insufficient to provide all birds an elevated resting place.

Pecking enrichment in the form of bales or pecking stones/pecking blocks is not generally provided in commercial broiler breeder houses, but could be helpful in fulfilling the need for exploration, and offer opportunities for the birds to perform a wider range of natural behaviours. In their review, Riber et al. (2017) evaluated different enrichments for broiler breeders. They concluded that potentially successful enrichments for broiler breeders were elevated resting places, cover panels and substrate (for broiler breeders housed in cage systems). However, they also concluded that further development of practical applicable enrichments is necessary, as there is little knowledge on the effect of the enrichments on behaviour and welfare, as well as their interaction with genotype and production system.

Transgenerational effects

Broiler breeders produce a large number of hatching eggs. This means that diseases or other factors during rearing and production in broiler breeder flocks may not only affect the egg production, egg quality and welfare of the breeder birds, but also the quality of the day-old chickens. Hygiene, to help prevent and protect against health issues, is therefore an important aspect of broiler breeder production. Moreover, there is increasing evidence that management of the breeder flock may have effects on performance, health and welfare of the progeny. A recent study that provided a low protein or a standard feed during rearing and production, showed that these two diets not only affected welfare of the breeders but also behaviour and learning capacity of the progeny (Li et al., 2018). Studies of laying hens indicate that stress in the breeder flock, via deposition of corticosterone in the egg, can affect fearfulness in the progeny. Management of broiler breeder flocks may thus not only be important for broiler breeder welfare, but also for the welfare of the final production broiler birds.

CHAPTER 2

Hatchery welfare

ANDY BUTTERWORTH AND INGRID DE JONG

Which came first – the welfare of the chicken, or the welfare of the egg?

Pedigree birds may have genetic influence over millions of final stage production birds. To enable this 'multiplication' – at each tier in the pyramid, fertile eggs are created by mating hen and cock, and these eggs are hatched in a semi-automated process within a building known as a hatchery. Hatcheries receive fertilised eggs, incubate them and then distribute day-old broiler chicks to the production farms. Hatcheries have become very large, with single hatcheries capable of producing over a million chicks per week. To enable this, the process has become highly automated with chicks being handled in large numbers, and in some countries and some companies, at high speed.

Fertile eggs arrive from the breeder farms – where the males and females have been kept and mated to produce fertile eggs. The 'quality' of the fertile eggs – their cleanliness (Figure 2.1), the absence of deformed, broken or cracked eggs, and the care with which they have

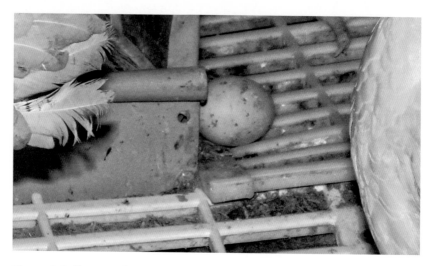

Figure 2.1 Eggs are fertilised and laid in the breeder farm. The hygiene of the egg is important – dirty eggs potentially carry infection to the hatchery – and 'floor eggs' – eggs not laid in the breeder farm nest – are often soiled with litter and faecal material.

been stored and transported, affects the hatching outcomes. Reijrink et al. (2008) note the extreme importance to the poultry business of the microenvironment during egg storage on the early incubation of chicks. In general, the longer eggs are stored (Figures 2.2 and 2.3), the lower their hatchability. Egg storage conditions are usually designed to optimise the humidity and temperature conditions to give the best egg storage and hatchability. Donofre et al. (2017) linked mechanical vibrations in the handling of eggs to the hatchability and quality of chicks. Torma and Kovácsné (2012) assessed the effects of mechanical impacts on hatchability of broiler breeders, and concluded that mechanical damage could adversely affect hatchability. The most direct metric of egg performance is hatchability – the percentage of fertilised eggs which progress to a healthy live chick. Typical hatchability rates are in the range from 82% to 90%, with the implication that between 18% and 10% of eggs were either not fertile, or did not develop into a viable chick.

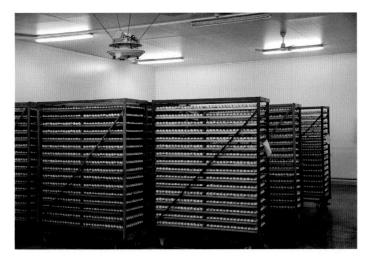

Figure 2.2 Eggs are stored on racks on arrival at the hatchery. Most hatcheries fumigate the eggs, often with formalin, at this stage – to reduce pathogen load on the shell surface.

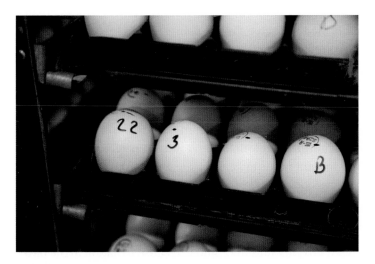

Figure 2.3 Eggs on a setter rack waiting to be placed in the setter, where they will be incubated for 18 days. In many countries – fertile hatching eggs must be marked – to prevent them entering the human food chain.

Because of the potential impacts on chick welfare, the RSPCA (2017) hatchery standards require that 'overall hatchability and the number of birds culled per day (including reason for culling) be monitored and recorded'.

Broiler chick incubation takes about 21 days, and is usually a two-step process. The first stage is incubation, carried out in setter chambers. Inside the setter, the eggs are placed on racks. Temperature and humidity are closely controlled, and air is circulated to provide oxygen and to help ensure uniform temperature. The eggs are tilted automatically and periodically on the racks to stop adhesion of the embryo to the inner shell membrane and to stimulate the development of the vasculosa (the blood vessel rich membrane which grows around the yolk). The eggs incubate in the setter for 18 days, and then are transferred from the egg racks to hatch trays, and to the hatcher chamber – where the chicks 'pip' (break through the eggshell) and hatch out in low flat trays. Many hatchery trays (or baskets) contain 180 eggs, and so about 180 chicks, but there are a number of designs of hatcher and of hatcher trays. During the hatch process, shell debris and fluff from the drying chicks creates an environment rich in shell and fluff debris (Figures 2.4 and 2.5).

To reduce 'contamination' and the risks of cross infection of chicks in the hatcher chamber, it has been usual practice to use disinfectant agents (Figure 2.6) (historically commonly formalin) to sanitise the air in the hatcher chamber during the hatch. The RSPCA (2017) hatchery standard, a standard which has quite comprehensive hatchery welfare requirements, identifies the welfare (and human health) risks of use of in-hatch formalin and other toxic disinfectants. When using a noxious substance, such as formalin, sanitation must be: performed only once in the hatcher; conducted when the majority of the birds are 'pipping' and not at peak emergence. This standard also notes that;

> Formalin is a noxious substance and can cause irritation to the bird's eyes and nasal passages, especially if used incorrectly. Consideration should be given to the use of alternative sanitisers, which are as effective but less noxious. (RSPCA, 2017, p. 4)

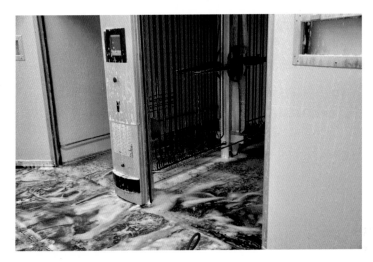

Figure 2.4 Setter and hatcher chambers are cleaned between batches. Hygiene is considered an important aspect of hatchery management because every single bird in the poultry 'chain' passes through hatcheries.

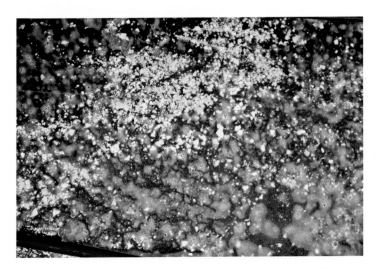

Figure 2.5 During the hatch, a lot of eggshell debris and fluff are generated, and there is significant risk of pathogen cross contamination of chicks by contact with, and inhalation of, this debris.

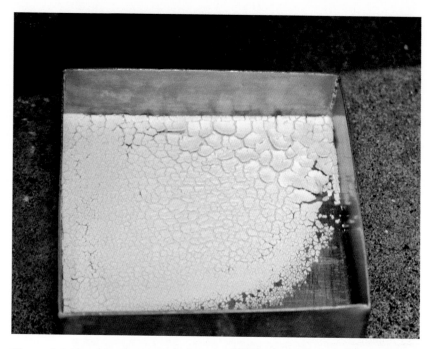

Figure 2.6 Formalin – evaporated into the air in the hatchery chamber to sanitise the air during the hatching process. Formalin is a noxious substance and can cause irritation to the bird's eyes and nasal passages (RSPCA, 2017).

The humidity and temperature conditions in the hatcher are regulated to provide the conditions required for hatching. Not all chicks hatch at the same time, the hatch is spread across a 'hatch window' (spread of hatch) with some chicks hatching within a short time of entering the hatching chamber, and some hatching only at the end of the hatching period. About 50% of chicks will hatch in the 10 hours in the middle of the hatch window, but chicks can differ in age by a whole day. The chicks are not 'fed or watered' during the hatch period – but they do not starve or become dehydrated, because they are able to utilise internal energy and liquid stores held in the residual yolk held in their bodies in the yolk sac. The yolk sac enables the hatchery process to function – the chicks can be hatched, sorted, vaccinated, sexed (if required), and then batched up for transport to the farms – without provision of food or water. However, there are time limits on how long the chick will tolerate absence of food and water, and this is one of the drivers of rapid handling and delivery to the farm.

Tong et al. (2015) investigated the effect of the time from hatch to removal from the hatcher chamber (pulling) by measuring plasma corticosterone in chicks with different durations of holding period. These authors concluded that shortening the hatch window and minimising the number of chicks that experience a long holding period would improve chick quality and physiological status, and this may be due to exposure to unfavourable environmental conditions during the holding period, that include relative feed and water deprivation. The total time between hatching and placement of the chickens in the broiler house may vary but is usually more than one day and can last up till 72 hours (Willemsen et al., 2010).

If the eggs hatch 'too early', the chicks are at risk of dehydration. If the eggs hatch 'too late', the result can be poor preparedness of the chicks for transport, and more live embryos in unhatched eggs. This increases the welfare risk that 'almost hatched' chicks which must be euthanised are not done so without delay, and hence humanely.

The factors that can affect the accuracy of the hatch window (Figure 2.7), and hence affect early chick welfare include: too short or too long an incubation period; poor control of setter humidity and temperature, or poor uniformity of temperature within the setter; insufficient ventilation; egg size greater or smaller than calculated for; use of eggs which have been stored for over-long periods (Figure 2.8) before setting; disease in the breeder birds resulting in disease in the incubating eggs.

A too long food and water deprivation period after hatch may result in increased mortality and impaired growth in the post-hatch period (Figure 2.9) (de Jong et al., 2017). Moreover, the food and water deprivation after hatch is considered a welfare issue, as chicks may show signs of dehydration and are thought to suffer from hunger after a relatively

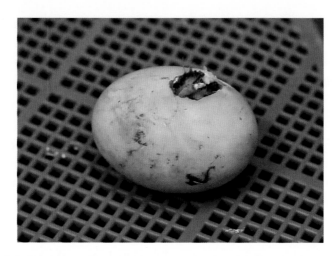

Figure 2.7 Chick hatching – the chick must pip (break) the eggshell from inside with the 'egg tooth' (a temporary hard tip to the beak). The process takes many hours, and not all chicks emerge at the same time – the hatch taking place across a hatch window of time.

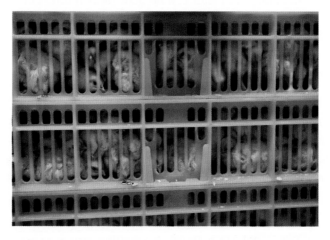

Figure 2.8 Chicks in a hatcher tray in a hatcher chamber. The environment is carefully controlled with respect to temperature and humidity. Disinfection agents (sometimes formalin vapour) are applied into the hatching chamber to 'clean' the chicks.

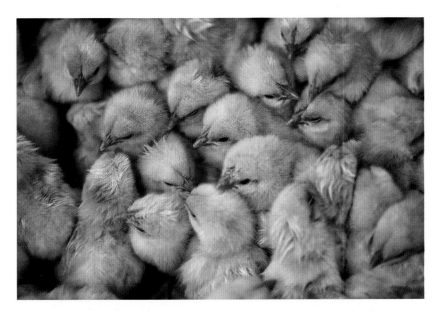

Figure 2.9 Chicks recently hatched in a hatcher tray. The chicks do not all hatch at exactly the same time, so some chicks can be several hours older than others. In most systems, no food or water is given – the chicks utilise energy and liquid in their yolk sacs.

long period in the hatcher, as can be the case for early hatched chickens. When day-old chicks start to eat, the intestines start to develop and it is thought that early post-hatch feeding may have positive effects on the welfare of broiler chickens as compared to the feed deprivation normally experienced in the hatcher (de Jong et al., 2017, 2018), although more research is necessary to further study these effects.

To overcome the welfare problems associated with post-hatch feed and water deprivation, systems have been developed (Figures 2.10 and 2.11) where chickens can either be fed in the hatchery, or hatch in the broiler house where they are able to reach food and water immediately after hatch. There are several commercially available systems for on-farm hatching, that differ in the degree of automation. However,

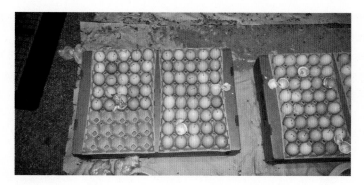

Figure 2.10 Example of a simple system for on-farm hatching. Eighteen-day incubated eggs are placed on cardboard trays and these are placed in the litter area of the broiler house. After hatching, the trays can be used as environmental enrichment for the broiler chickens or removed from the broiler house.

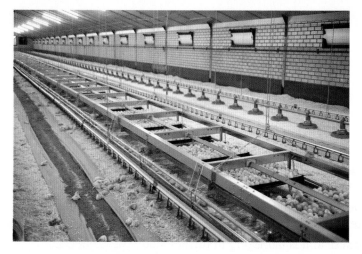

Figure 2.11 Example of a system for on-farm hatching that requires less farmer labour as compared to the cardboard boxes. Eighteen-day incubated eggs are placed on special setter trays that are placed on a rail system in the broiler houses. After hatching, chickens fall on a rubber belt and will dry. After drying they will move to the edge of the belt and fall in the litter, where they can access feed and water. After use, the setters and remaining eggshells will be removed and disinfected. The rail system can then be lifted to the ceiling.

these systems are not suitable for each broiler farmer and broiler house. Heating systems must be able to heat the house to temperatures suitable for hatching chickens, and the hatching process involves more labour for the farmer such as recording egg shell temperatures to monitor the hatching process and identifying and culling second-grade chicks, and removing eggshells from the house.

Dealing with unwanted chicks

On day 21, when the chicks have hatched, the chicks are removed from the hatcher chamber, and then are inspected. Small, partially hatched, deformed or sick chicks (so-called second-grade chicks) are removed. The humane destruction of such chicks and also of nearly partially developed and almost hatched chicks 'in shell' must be accomplished with care and using methods that cause immediate death. Hatcheries are equipped with systems that ensure humane euthanisation of second-grade chicks. In many instances this is achieved by use of a high-speed macerator capable of destroying chicks in a very short time frame (less than 100 ms) and which ensure that the entire chick is destroyed with no risk of recovery. Although not a pleasant business, the killing of sick or damaged chicks takes place in every hatchery – and should be carried out in a rapid, careful and effective way. Methods recommended by the RSPCA are: (1) instantaneous mechanical destruction (maceration); (2) exposure to a maximum of 2% oxygen by volume and 90% argon (or other inert gas) by volume in atmospheric air; (3) exposure to a maximum of 30% carbon dioxide by volume and a minimum of 60% argon (or other inert gas) by volume in atmospheric air, with no more than 2% residual oxygen.

Use of 100% carbon dioxide gas is not permitted as a method of disposing of birds by the RSPCA. All methods should ensure that individual chicks are rapidly and humanely killed (Figure 2.12), and that sick or compromised chicks do not 'wait' to be culled, for example, by waiting to be collected in a group in a tray, but are killed humanely as soon as is possible (Figure 2.13).

With on-farm hatching, such a system should also be present on the farm to ensure humane killing of sick or malformed chicks.

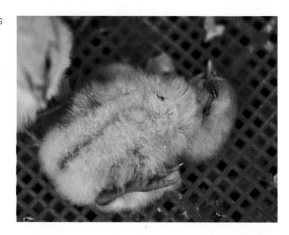

Figure 2.12 Some chicks will be sick, deformed or damaged, and should be euthanised without delay using a humane method.

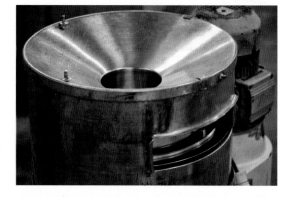

Figure 2.13 Portable macerator. Although not a pleasant business, the killing of sick or damaged chicks takes place in every hatchery – and should be carried out in a rapid, careful and effective way to help ensure best possible welfare.

Effects of automation

The degree of automation varies between hatcheries. Broiler chicks are produced in very large numbers – about 900 million in the UK, about 50 billion globally annually. Because of the large numbers of animals involved, and the high throughputs in individual hatcheries, automation is a common feature of hatcheries in the developed world. In countries where throughputs of birds may not be so high, and where labour costs are lower, manual handling systems are still important in hatcheries.

Separation from eggshell waste

Chicks are taken from the hatching chamber in trays, and then separated from the eggshell waste by an egg separator, which tips the chicks onto a series of rollers that separate live chicks from unhatched eggs and eggshell debris. The slight, but potential, risk of automated chick separation is that live chicks fail to be sorted effectively by the rollers and enter the machine which handles the eggshell waste. Egg shell waste must be treated as if it 'by default' contains live animals, as unhatched eggs which may contain almost hatched chicks will also be present in the shell waste. For this reason, eggshell waste, and unhatched eggs), should be immediately passed through a high-speed macerator of sufficient speed and precision to cause the immediate destruction and death of any living chicks or in shell embryos. To ensure this, the macerator must be (1) of sufficient capacity, (2) of design to prevent build-up of material before maceration occurs – to ensure that any live animals pass immediately into the macerator without 'piling up' in waste debris, and (3) must be maintained, inspected and checked to ensure rapid effective action. The RSPCA (2017, p. 5) hatchery standard recognises these risks and requires that:

> Where automatic sorters are used, the following conditions must be satisfied: the tipping of birds from the hatcher trays must be

gradual and ensure that birds are delivered directly onto the sorting equipment; birds must be protected from falling from the sides of the sorter or falling into the debris; empty hatcher trays must be examined thoroughly for any remaining birds or unhatched eggs prior to washing.

After separation, the chicks are usually moved around the hatchery on belt systems. The technology of belts is very similar to that used for moving fruit and food products in factories, and much of the equipment is either modified food processing equipment or is very similar in design to factory processing machinery. The use of established automated processing technology creates both possible benefits and potential risks to the chicks.

Sorting and counting

If companies require 'sexed' chicks – then, after an initial 'grading' to remove obviously sick or deformed chicks – the chicks are then taken by a moving belt to a carousel, or to a long sorting belt. Here the chicks are picked up individually and sexed using feather patterns and feather colours. The males and females are passed by the operator into separate chutes, or belts for the males and females. If 'as hatched' (mixed sex) chicks are required at the farm, then the carousel or sorting belt is bypassed. Many broiler farms rear both males and females, and thus 'as hatched' chickens, but sexing is universally carried out in laying hen farming. If needle vaccination is required (this is more common for breeder bird chicks and for laying hens), then the chicks are picked up individually by hand and injected subcutaneously by placing them against the surface of a machine which locates the bird and injects the vaccine. This is a skilled process and the positioning and handling of the chick is critical to avoid damage, and to ensure effective vaccination – and this is carried out at high speed and with high rates of repetition by the hatchery operatives.

After sexing (and any required injection vaccination, which may alternatively take place after counting into baskets) the next stage is usually for the chicks to be counted into trays or baskets. In order to allow individual chicks to be 'seen' by the counters, the chicks are passed onto a series of increasingly narrow and faster-moving belts (called accelerator belts) until they have been spread out into single file, and at higher velocity. The counter can register individual chicks in this single file, and as they pass into the basket they are counted, and the basket moved on, or a deflector plate moved, to separate the chicks into counted batches in the trays. The trays usually carry 40 or 60 chicks per tray (but there are many designs). Abeyesinghe et al. (2001) demonstrated that chicks show significant behavioural responses to vibration and motions. Svedberg (1996, 1997, 1998) evaluated chick separators and chick counters as individual components of the system, and Svedberg (1997, 1998) assessed one type of chick separator (RRAL-200) used in Sweden, with regard to welfare impacts. The conclusions of these studies were that, if the machines were carefully set up and adjusted to chick size, and were monitored, maintained and adjusted in use, if required, then the use of these machines could be acceptable. Svedberg concluded that the adjustments required to minimise damage to the chicks included minimisation of the total and cumulative height from which chicks fell and ensuring that the belts and tracks were designed so that chicks could not fall from the transport surfaces, or become caught and trapped in the mechanisms.

Vaccination

As the chicks move along the belts in the trays they are usually then vaccinated by spray (aerosol). Laying hen chicks are often subjected to additional manual subcutaneous vaccination at some point within the system. The chicks receive a relatively small volume of vaccination in the aerosol mist spray, but are 'wetted' by this process, and must be protected from chilling in the minutes following spray vaccination. Nääs et al. (2014) assessed factors affecting heat loss in 1 day-old pullets inside a hatchery and concluded that temperature control was important to protect young chicks from both chilling and overheating during hatchery handling processes.

Accelerations and decelerations/impacts

Knowles et al. (2004) measured accelerations (and decelerations) as chicks moved through automated hatchery equipment by using Tinytag data loggers (Gemini Data Loggers UK Ltd). Knowles et al. (2004) demonstrated a very clear relationship between a chick's ability to stand and changes in velocity of greater than 0.4 m/s. Above this speed, over 80% of birds were not able to stand. Stability of speed change (that is, fewer accelerations and decelerations) were noted to be the most critical factor for overall time spent standing.

Svedberg (1996, 1997) found, in post-mortem examinations, subcutaneous haemorrhages on the side of the head in some chicks subjected to high-speed counter accelerations in poorly set up counters. Both Knowles et al. (2004) and Svedberg (1996, 1997, 1998) conclude that significant improvements in welfare outcomes for chicks can be achieved by observant assessment of what actually happens to the chicks in the automated systems, and through implementation of careful machine adjustments.

Righting time and orientation

During their progression through the hatchery system, chicks fall (Figure 2.14) and are tumbled (Figure 2.15) and rolled by the action and speed of the belts (Figures 2.16 and 2.17). The chicks also impact surfaces – sometimes after falls from distances of multiples of their own height – and at these times they impact surfaces or deflector plates. Knowles et al. (2004) analysed the time it took for chicks to right themselves (re-establish stable upright posture), and this metric was used as a measure of the degree and duration of disorientation of the chicks.

The same authors examined the orientation of chicks as they passed through the automated system by video analysis. 'Disorientation' was measured calculating the percentage of chicks that were not on their feet in time-selected video frames. The gradient at which the belts rose

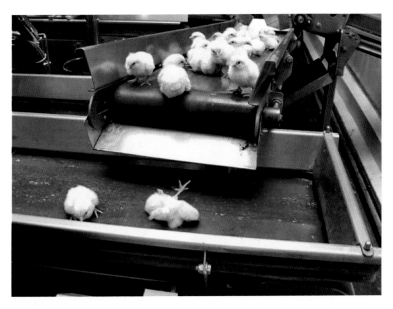

Figure 2.14 Chicks dropping from a belt surface at a junction between two belts.

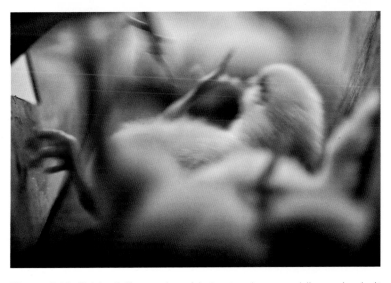

Figure 2.15 Chicks falling and unable to stand on a rapidly moving belt.

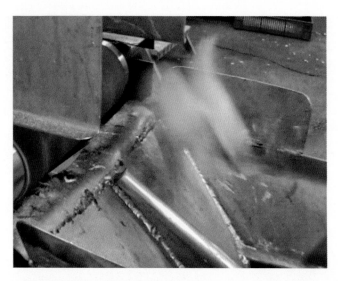

Figure 2.16 Chicks being passed at high speed into baskets after being accelerated past an electronic counter.

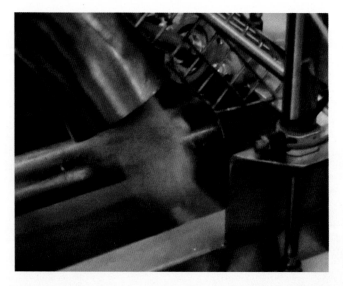

Figure 2.17 High-speed contact with surfaces at junctions and in counters like this present both physical and pathogen contamination risks to the chicks.

or descended was noted by Knowles et al. (2004) as affecting the ability of chicks to remain on their feet. The RSPCA (2017, p. 6) hatchery standards recognise the importance of the automated machinery in hatcheries and require:

> Where automatic conveyor belt systems are used, these must: be designed to ensure that birds cannot become trapped, provide adequate side protection to contain the birds. (Hnd 1.8) Where necessary, additional side protection must be fitted to the conveyor belt system to ensure the wellbeing of the birds. The design and speed of the automatic conveyor belt must not cause injuries to the birds.

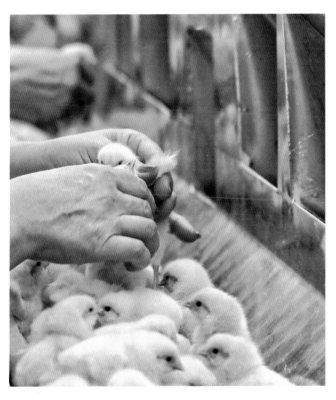

Figure 2.18 Sexing broiler chicks using wing feather patterns.

It is very apparent, from personal experience and from published work, that the severity of the impact of handling on newly hatched chicks varies very much between hatcheries. Some hatcheries remain very 'manual', and, even in highly automated hatcheries, there are still quite a lot of human handling tasks – moving trolleys of eggs and chicks, grading, sexing, some forms of vaccination. For all manual tasks (Figure 2.18), the care, skill and consideration of the humans will be an important part of chick welfare. For highly automated systems, there is scope for damage to chicks by the automated systems. Svedberg (1996, 1997, 1998), Knowles et al. (2004), and reductions to the absolute practical minimum of height of drops, rates of acceleration and deceleration, use and design of high-speed accelerators for counting, the incline angle of vertical belts, the hygiene of belts and surfaces, and a reduction in the number of changes of direction (corners) and impact surfaces (which sometimes have specifically designed deflector plates, but avoidance of the need to 'deflect' would be better) will probably have quite significant (and even measurable) improving effects on the experience of the chicks in the handling system, on their welfare, and even potentially on their health. The chicks usually arrive on the farm within 24 hours of hatch, but sometimes they may be sent on longer journeys – sometimes transported by air, and then the journey times can be prolonged.

With on-farm hatching, this handling and processing of chickens is absent. This is one of the reasons that these systems are considered as having welfare benefits as compared to conventional hatching.

Hygiene

Every chick in an automated hatchery passes over belt and other handling surfaces (Figure 2.19). The hygiene and material of the surfaces have the potential to increase the exposure of chicks to faecal contamination from other chicks, and hence pathogens. Butterworth et al. (2001) found associations between typed strains of *Staphylococcus aureus* and

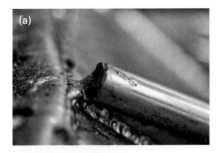

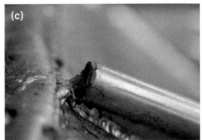

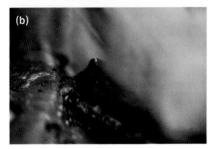

Figure 2.19 (a) A dirty surface close up; (b) a chick falls across the surface; (c) the surface is clean, the chick is contaminated.

Escherichia coli isolated from bone and joint lesions in lame broilers, and the same strains identified in hatcheries.

This suggests that it may be possible to reduce exposure to infection by improving hygiene at these critical points and by reducing the impact, rolling and contact of chicks with deflector plates and surfaces. The lack of inter-processing cleaning of belt surfaces in most plants during the hatching and handling of chicks, which may be a period of seven hours, may mean that *S. aureus*, particularly, has a prolonged window of opportunity for contact with chicks.

Hatcheries have the potential to disseminate pathogens because they are at the centre of the poultry production chain. Casadio et al. (2014) evaluated the level of bacterial contamination of eggs and dead-in-shell chicks, and the possible involvement of hatcheries in spread of haemolytic antimicrobial resistant *E. coli*. Osman et al. (2018) also looked at the role of hatcheries in bacterial pathogen contamination. These authors found that the β-lactam resistance gene could be found in antimicrobial resistant (AMR) *E. coli* from chicks from multiple breeder flocks, suggesting that hatcheries could be a reservoir, or 'distributor' of antimicrobial resistant *E. coli*, posing a potential threat to poultry and human health. Osman et al. (2018) examined the role of *E. coli* as one of the major bacterial contaminants of poultry hatcheries. They found that the bacterial contamination of eggshells at arrival was rather low. However, at hatching, the bacterial contamination was significantly increased. These authors highlight how the hatchery may act to amplify the effect of bacterial contamination. As an example, *Pseudomonas aeruginosa* and *E. coli* were found in 5% and 10% of the batches of arriving eggs, respectively, but were then found in 15% and 100% of dead-in-shell chicks at hatching. The RSPCA (2017, p. 1) standards recognise the importance of hygiene in disease control and chick welfare, stating 'All surfaces and equipment within the hatchery must be: a) maintained in good condition b) cleaned regularly.'

Chicks on the floor

Chicks which fall from the automated handling system onto the floor are a welfare problem as they can become lost under machinery or may remain on the floor for a period of time until they are detected and either returned to the handling system, or euthanised. A simple metric of 'handling quality' is whether (and how many) chicks are observed on the floor.

Light

Conventional hatching involves keeping eggs in darkness until they hatch and then providing low levels of light for early hatched chicks. In 'in hatchery feeding' systems the chicks are provided with light. Studies, such as those of Archer (2017), indicate that light provided during incubation can affect welfare, including fear responses in later life. This area requires further study, but there is increasing attention to provision of light during parts of the incubation period, as well as during handling. In many parts of the world it is common to illuminate chicks under blue lighting (Figure 2.20) during sorting, handling and while waiting for delivery. The logic of using blue light is not entirely clear – as it is known that birds have high sensitivity to blue light having four receptors (mammals have three) of which one receptor is most specifically sensitive in the violet and ultraviolet parts of the light spectrum.

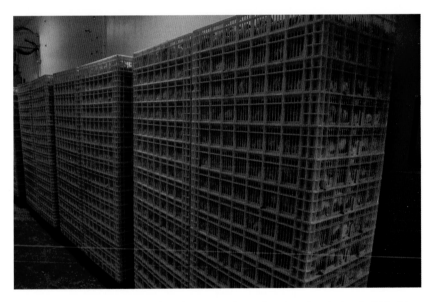

Figure 2.20 Chicks in their hatcher trays just after hatch – being held in blue light.

CHAPTER 3

Influences of housing and management on broiler welfare

JOY MENCH, INGRID DE JONG AND ANDY BUTTERWORTH

Broiler housing

Housing and management during grow out are obviously key factors influencing the welfare of broiler chickens. Broilers can experience good welfare in a range of housing systems – providing that the birds are genetically suited to that particular system, and that the system is well managed to achieve the desired welfare outcomes. In this chapter, we will first describe the different broiler housing systems, and then discuss aspects of management that are most critical to achieving good broiler welfare.

In Europe and the Americas, broiler chickens are managed in three general types of systems: (1) fully indoors (Figure 3.1a); (2) mainly indoors but given access to the outdoors (free-range); (3) mainly outdoors (Figure 3.1b) but provided with a structure or house in which the birds can be confined at night and during inclement weather (pastured). Most large-scale commercial production takes place in fully indoor systems, although the popularity of free-range broiler production, and pastured broiler production to a lesser extent, is growing in some countries. This appears to be due mainly to an increased demand for animals produced outdoors in general, as is the case in parts of the EU (the Netherlands, Germany and the UK), and for organic foods, with organic certification programmes requiring that birds be given outdoor access.

In fully indoor systems, about 20,000–30,000 broilers are reared in a house on an all-litter floor. The birds are placed in the house as soon as they are transported there from the hatchery; they are then grown there to the desired market weight. Feed and water are delivered automatically. Nipple watering systems are typically used in order to minimise problems with water spillage and consequently wet litter. Houses may either have tunnel ventilation or be naturally ventilated, depending upon the local climate. Free-range production houses are often similar to those used for fully indoor rearing, except that outdoor access is provided to the birds via pop holes in the house that can be opened. The outdoor area can either be a small porch/veranda (usually enclosed by wire but covered to provide shade and protection from overhead predators) or a larger range/pasture area.

Pastured systems are more variable in design than fully indoor or free-range systems. Flock sizes in pastured systems are much smaller (usually around 1000–2000 birds) and pastured producers typically raise slower-growing or dual-purpose breeds, which are more suitable for outdoor rearing. There are two main types of pastured systems: day-out and day-in. In day-out systems, the broilers are free to roam on the range during the day once they are old enough to be well-feathered, although they are enclosed in a structure at night for protection from predators

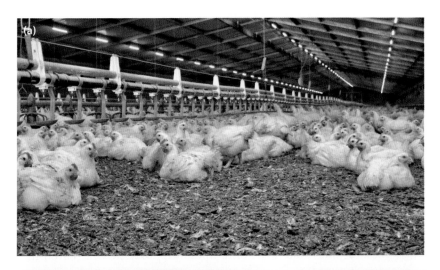

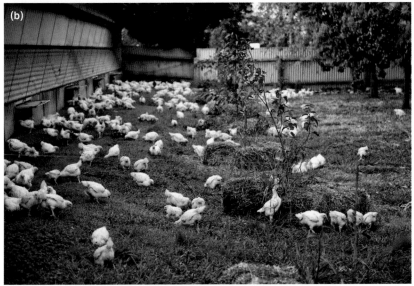

Figure 3.1 Examples of broiler housing systems: (a) fully indoor and (b) provided with a free range.

(and in which they can also be enclosed in inclement weather). In day-in systems, the broilers are kept enclosed throughout rearing in a floorless structure that can be moved around the range. The broilers can therefore forage on the pasture underneath the structure but are kept in an enclosure that can be protected (for example by being covered with a tarpaulin) at night, in inclement weather or during the brooding stage.

Each of these systems will have particular risks and benefits for broiler welfare. However, to support good welfare, all systems should be designed and maintained to prevent injury to the birds, provide them with opportunities to express their normal behaviours, allow adequate biosecurity, and minimise exposure of birds to hazards, contaminants and stressors – like loud noise or temperature extremes.

Cage rearing systems are also being marketed for broiler chickens, although they are currently used on a commercial scale mainly in Russia, the Middle East and Asia, especially China (Shields and Greger, 2013). These systems are comprised of large (colony) cages, housing between 80 and 200 broilers per cage, arranged in multiple tiers (Figure 3.2). Feeding, watering, and manure removal are automated, and the cage floor is made of soft plastic mesh or a belt that is covered in litter. Broiler behaviour is restricted in these cages compared to the systems described above, and they are only allowed in the EU if they are designed so as to provide the birds with continuous access to litter (Council Directive 2007/43/EC). The major welfare advantage of cages is related to bird handling prior to processing, which involves a risk for injuries (fractures, bruises). In some systems, the cage floor slides out and the birds drop onto a belt that moves them to the loading area, while in others the entire cage module is removed and loaded onto the truck for transport to the processing area. Both methods eliminate the need for people (or machines) to catch birds for loading. Because there has been little published scientific research on the behaviour or health of broilers in the newer colony cage systems, our discussion about management will focus on loose housing systems.

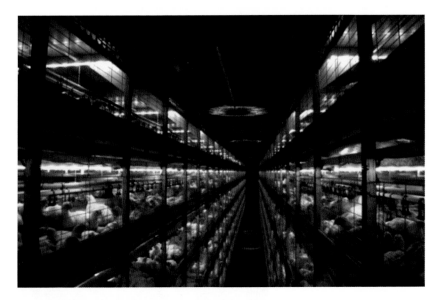

Figure 3.2 Example of cage based broiler housing system.

Key management factors

Litter

Litter plays an important role in maintaining good animal welfare in broiler housing systems (Figure 3.3). Litter:

- dilutes manure and therefore reduces contact between the birds and their faeces
- absorbs excess moisture from droppings and drinkers and promotes drying by increasing the surface area of the floor
- cushions the floor surface, which is typically earth or concrete, and thus provides a more comfortable standing and lying surface for the birds
- provides a layer of insulation that protects the birds from being excessively cooled by the floor surface

- is used by the birds for performing two important behaviours, foraging (ground-scratching and ground-pecking) and dustbathing (a grooming behaviour that involves the birds working loose material through their feathers in order to remove excess oils).

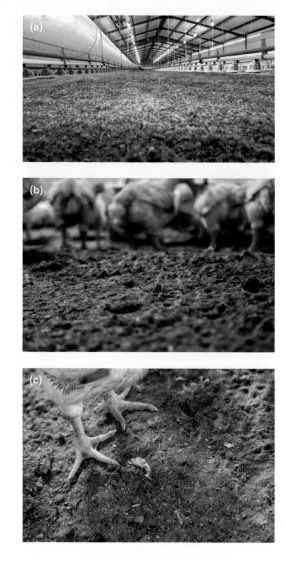

Figure 3.3 Various litter conditions in the broiler house: (a) new substrate; (b) wet and sticky; (c) wet and compacted.

However, litter is also a potential source of welfare problems. Litter that is too dry generates excessive dust that can cause respiratory problems, while litter that is too wet is a major risk factor for contact dermatitis (hock burns and footpad dermatitis) (de Jong et al., 2012; Chapter 4, this book). Wet litter produces excessive ammonia, which is a respiratory, ocular and skin irritant, and also fosters the growth of toxin-producing fungi that can cause serious health problems. Pathogenic organisms can proliferate in contaminated, poorly maintained litter, including the organisms that cause avian influenza, Gumboro disease, laryngotracheitis, bronchitis and coccidiosis (Ritz et al., 2017). Litter that is so wet that it becomes caked (clumped) cannot be used by the birds for foraging or dustbathing, and it also does not provide a surface that is suitable for resting or thermal insulation.

The health impacts of poor litter condition affect not only welfare but also production costs. For example, Ritz et al. (2017) conservatively estimated that poor litter condition in US broiler flocks costs the industry US$950 per 20,000 bird flock, due to lower feed conversion, increased incidence of disease and parasites, and increased condemnations and downgrades, including those due to breast blisters.

The key, then, is to provide a sufficient quantity of well-maintained litter to confer the desired welfare benefits while reducing risks to health. A wide variety of materials can be used as litter. These include wood shavings/sawdust, wood chips or bark, rice hulls, peanut hulls, peat, sand, crushed corn cobs, chopped straw or hay, and processed paper. The type of litter material chosen by a producer typically depends upon cost and availability, although materials can differ in their moisture-holding capacity and hence may require different types and standards of management. Studies comparing the effects of different litter materials on the incidence of contact dermatitis are summarised in de Jong et al. (2012). In general, however, what is important is to maintain the moisture content of whatever litter is used at about 20–35% (Pastor, 2016; Ritz et al., 2017). This is mainly achieved by ventilation and house temperature control, and by diagnosing and correcting causes of wet litter, including leaking or poorly adjusted drinkers and poor concrete floor construction. Regular assessment of litter quality on farms is critical (Welfare Quality, 2009; de Jong et al., 2012), since once litter becomes caked it is difficult to correct the problem.

A variety of factors besides litter type can affect litter moisture. These include weather conditions (especially humid, wet and cold weather), use of foggers and evaporative coolers during hot weather, spillage or leakage from drinkers, and high stocking densities. Because about 80% of the water broilers drink is excreted, higher levels of nutrients that increase water intake (for example, sodium, magnesium) can also cause wet litter. For example, a 1% increase in the protein content of the diet increases water consumption (and excretion) by about 3% (Alleman and Leclercq, 1997). Water excretion can similarly be increased if gut health is impaired, for example in birds infected with *E. coli*, *Campylobacter* spp., or Coccidia.

As required by the Council Directive (2007/43/EC), in the EU litter is cleaned out and replaced with clean litter between each flock. In the USA (and some other major broiler producing countries like Brazil), litter is typically re-used for some period of time, generally 1 or 2 years (Hess et al., 2009). Reasons for re-use of litter include environmental regulations restricting the use of litter as fertiliser and local scarcity of unused litter material. There is evidence that re-use of litter can be beneficial to broiler health, as long as there have not been serious disease problems in the flocks previously raised on that litter. Placing young broilers on used litter exposes them to various microorganisms and can help to inoculate them against common pathogens and establish a gut 'flora' (Lee et al., 2011; Wang et al., 2016). Before introducing a new flock, caked litter is removed. The litter to be re-used is then treated to reduce ammonia and bacterial and viral loads (Ritz et al., 2017). This can be accomplished either by composting the litter *in situ*, or by adding chemical or biological amendments (that is, acidifying agents, odour/ammonia absorbents, microbial/enzymatic inhibitors) to it. A top dressing of new litter may also be applied to the re-used litter.

Air quality

It is critical to maintain good air quality in indoor environments for broilers (de Jong et al., 2012). Air quality includes the thermal environment (temperature and humidity), and pollutants such as particulate matter ('dust'), and gases (for example, ammonia, carbon monoxide). Failure to maintain air quality within acceptable limits will result in flock health problems. The major mechanism for maintaining good air quality in commercial broiler houses is ventilation.

Thermal environment

House temperature is affected by seasonal factors, stocking density and ventilation rate. The recommended temperatures for broilers decrease progressively from the first day of life; the primary breeders' management manuals provide information about the appropriate temperature ranges for different genetic stocks of broilers throughout rearing. The behaviour of the birds can be used to assess thermal conditions. They will huddle together when they are too cold, and pant and show behavioural changes (reduced activity, reduced feeding, alignment with air flows) to dissipate heat, or to reduce internal metabolic heat generation, when they are too hot. Older, fast-growing, broilers are particularly susceptible to heat stress because of their high rate of metabolic heat production. House humidity is affected by outside humidity, stocking density, ventilation rate, bird liveweight, indoor temperature, drinker type and management, and water consumption and spillage (de Jong et al., 2012). Humidity lower than 50% leads to an increase in dust and can thus make the birds more susceptible to respiratory disease. Humidity higher than 70% after the first few days of life causes wet litter and can lead to birds being thermally uncomfortable if the temperature is also high. Some producers use water misting systems to temporarily reduce house temperatures. However, misting systems also increase house humidity, and so cannot be used as long-term moderators of high house temperature.

Air pollutants

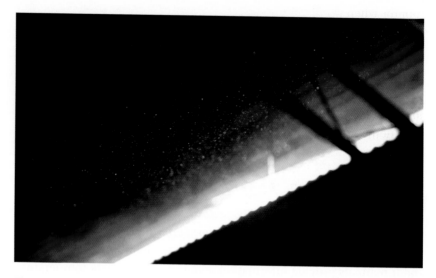

Figure 3.4 Dust in a poultry house made visible in a beam of light.

Ammonia and dust are the two primary air pollutants in broiler houses. Ammonia originates from the decomposition of manure in the litter. The most important factors affecting ammonia production are air temperature, ventilation rate, humidity, feed composition, age of the litter, litter pH and moisture content, litter type, stocking density, and bird age (Al-Homidan et al., 2003). High concentrations of ammonia in the litter can cause skin lesions like hock burn and footpad dermatitis. High concentrations of ammonia in the air can cause changes in the respiratory tract that impair respiratory function and make the birds susceptible to respiratory infection, including loss of cilia in the trachea, increased mucus secretion, and lesions of the air sacs (Anderson et al., 1966; Oyetunde et al., 1978). High ammonia levels can also cause eye inflammation and corneal damage (Aziz, 2010). Broilers find ammonia aversive, and if given a choice will avoid concentrations of ammonia above 20 ppm (Jones et al., 2005). In general, it is recommended that ammonia levels be kept at less than 20–25 ppm at bird height, but it may be difficult to achieve these levels in commercial houses, particularly during colder months when ventilation rates need to be decreased to maintain comfortable air temperatures in the house (David et al., 2015b).

Dust in broiler houses is composed of litter material, feathers and feather follicles, skin scales, feed, and inorganic particles (from building materials) (Figure 3.4). Dust particles vary in size. The ones of most concern for broiler welfare are the smaller, respirable, particles, which can cause irritation of the trachea and damage to the mucus membranes and lung by being inhaled deep into the lung and air sacs. Inhaled dust can carry harmful bacteria, viruses and toxins produced by fungi and bacteria (endotoxins) into the lungs (David et al., 2015a). Factors affecting dust levels include the quality and type of litter, bird activity, temperature, humidity and ventilation rate.

Lighting

Poultry are extremely light-sensitive. They absorb light not only through their eyes but also through their skulls, where the light stimulates parts of the brain to produce hormones controlling growth and reproduction. For that reason, light management is an important aspect of broiler production. Broiler chicks are usually exposed to continuous bright light for the first few days of life to facilitate them finding food and water. Thereafter, a lighting programme is imposed with the aim of optimising production (Figure 3.5).

Light has four elements: photoperiod (the durations of light and dark periods in a 24-hour cycle), intensity (brightness), source, and spectrum (the mixture of different colours in the light). The effects of these different elements on broiler welfare are reviewed in de Jong et al. (2012). However, these elements cannot easily be considered separately because they interact with one another. To complicate matters, a variety of photoperiods and light sources are used by the commercial industry, and photoperiods and light intensities in a flock may be modified a number of times as the birds age.

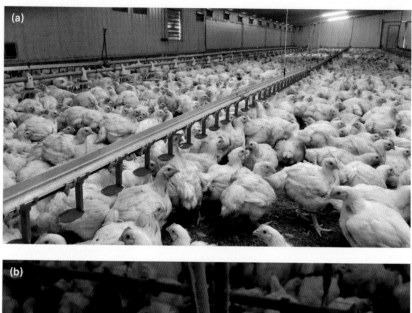

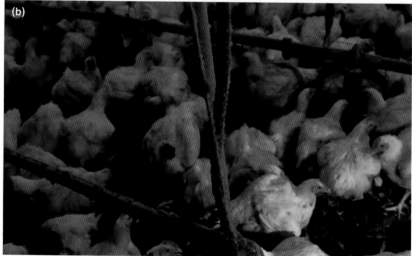

Figure 3.5 Birds at different light levels: (a) about 50 lux, approximately 5 foot candles; (b) about 5 lux, approximately 0.5 foot candles.

From the perspective of animal welfare, lighting should achieve a number of goals, including giving broilers distinct periods of rest and activity; stimulating their normal behaviours like dustbathing; allowing them to see well enough to access feed and water, utilise other features of their environment (that is, enrichments if provided) and engage in normal social interactions with other birds in the flock; and promoting good health and physical condition (for example, good musculoskeletal condition and feathering). There is no single 'ideal' lighting programme, but there is evidence that some aspects of lighting programmes that have been used in commercial production have consistently negative effects on welfare (de Jong et al., 2012). Broilers raised under continuous or near-continuous photoperiods, without an adequate dark period, have higher rates of health problems, including sudden death syndrome, spiking mortality, tibial dyschondroplasia, eye enlargement and leg problems. Light intensities below 5 lux are associated with eye enlargement, poorer gait scores and more footpad dermatitis (Deep et al., 2013; Yang et al., 2018). It is also important for there to be a sufficient intensity contrast between the light and dark periods in order for the birds in the flock to show synchronised rhythms of rest and activity (Alvino et al., 2009). The EU broiler directive (Council Directive 2007/43/EC) requires that there be light levels of at least 20 lux illuminating at least 80% of the usable area of the house, and that light must follow a 24 hour rhythm from 1 week of age until 3 days before slaughter, with a dark period of at least 6 hours total each 24 hours and an uninterrupted dark period of at least 4 hours.

A potentially important shift that is occurring now is the increasing use of light emitting diode (LED) lighting sources in broiler houses for energy efficiency. Unlike fluorescent and incandescent lighting, LED lighting can be adjusted to provide a variety of light spectra. The peak of spectral sensitivity is similar in poultry and humans. However, birds have four spectrally distinct cone pigments derived from the protein opsin, whereas mammals have only three cone pigments. As a consequence, poultry are likely to be more sensitive to red and blue light than humans (Lewis and Morris, 2000). Poultry can also see into the ultraviolet range, a range that is invisible to humans, although further study is required to determine if there are welfare implications of this for farmed poultry. Poultry feathers reflect ultraviolet wavelengths, and this presumably provides some kind of social information to other birds. Fluorescent and incandescent lights do not provide ultraviolet wavelengths, but full-spectrum LED lights are now available for use in poultry facilities, and these provide a lighting environment that mimics sunlight and that could potentially improve broiler welfare (James et al., 2018).

Stocking density

Stocking densities can vary from one flock to another based on a number of factors, including seasonal variations in temperature and humidity, bird genetics and desired market-age body weight (Figure 3.6). Under the EU broiler directive (Council Directive 2007/43/EC), the maximum stocking density allowed is 33 kg body weight/m^2 of floor space unless certain environmental conditions can be met, in which case the maximum density can be up to 39 kg/m^2. Stocking density can be further increased to up to 42 kg/m^2 if the environmental standards are met *and* if mortality and other specified health measures do not indicate reduced welfare. A 2017 survey (European Commission, 2018) showed that 34% of EU broilers were kept at densities up to 33 kg/m^2, 40% were kept at densities between 34 and 39 kg/m^2, and 26% were kept at densities between 39 and 42 kg/m^2.

The US does not have federal regulatory standards for keeping broilers, but many broiler producers follow the guidelines established by the industry's trade organisation, the National Chicken Council (NCC) (2017). Broilers are marketed at a wider range of body weights in the USA than in Europe, with small broilers (around 1 kg liveweight) marketed as whole birds called Cornish game hens, and the largest broilers, weighing between 3.4 and 4.1 kg and marketed between 7 and 9 weeks

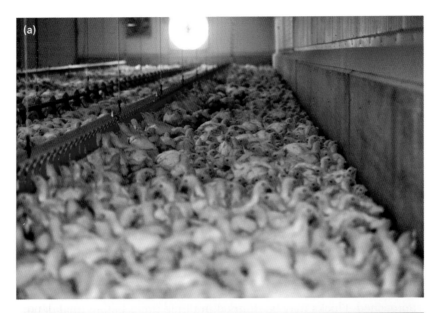

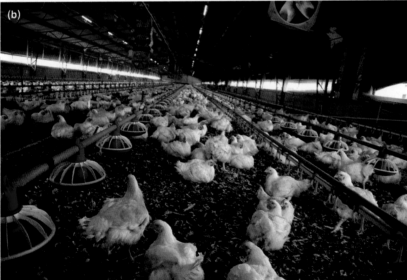

Figure 3.6 (a) High stocking density (approximately 44 kg/m²); (b) lower stocking density (approximately 28 kg/m²).

of age, normally grown for the further-processed products market (for example, sausages, chicken nuggets); the average market weight of a broiler in the USA is 2.8 kg (NCC, 2018). The NCC suggests different maximum stocking densities for different weight categories of birds, ranging from 32 kg/m^2 for birds with a market weight of less than 2 kg up to 44 kg/m^2 for birds with a market weight of more than 3.4 kg.

Stocking density ranges in the EU and USA are therefore similar. However, a difference that affects the amount of space available to the birds during the late stages of production relates to how the stocking density is achieved. In the USA, broilers are stocked initially at the density appropriate to their target body weight, meaning that the final density is actually lower as a result of mortality. In some countries in Europe, however, birds are initially stocked at a higher density (number of birds per unit area), and then a proportion of the flock is removed ('thinning') when the target stocking density (bird weight per unit area) is approached. Flocks may be thinned multiple times before final depopulation. Thinning has raised bird welfare concerns, since it involves withdrawal of food and water, as well as disruption of the flock due to catching of the birds being thinned (Dawkins, 2018). There are also potential biosecurity risks associated with this practice.

Many studies have evaluated the effects of stocking density on broiler welfare, with the aim of determining an acceptable maximum stocking density (de Jong et al., 2012; Dawkins, 2018). A variety of welfare outcomes have been assessed in these studies, including mortality, growth rate, indicators of physiological stress, fearfulness, behavioural restriction, behavioural disturbance, space use and preferences, and pathology. Overall these studies show that welfare can be negatively affected at higher stocking densities, with decreases in growth rate and walking ability and increased hock burn, footpad dermatitis and skin scratches seen as stocking density increases. In addition, studies of space use and preference indicate that broilers seem to prefer stocking densities lower than the maximum density allowed under the EU broiler directive (Council Directive 2007/43/EC). However, there is no clear 'cutoff' point that applies to all measures or all housing situations. What appears to be more important than density *per se* is that producers are able to maintain good thermal, air quality and litter condition in the house under higher stocking density conditions. It is for this reason that the EU broiler directive allows higher stocking densities if:

- the ammonia level in the house is maintained at 20 ppm or less
- the carbon dioxide level in the house is maintained at 3000 ppm or less
- the inside temperature is maintained so as not to exceed the outside temperature by more than 3°C
- the average relative humidity inside the house over a 48 hour period does not exceed 70% when the outside temperature is below 10°C. (Council Directive 2007/43/EC)

In addition to maintaining good environmental and litter condition, producers need to regularly monitor aspects of broiler health to ensure that broilers are not overstocked. In a recent survey of EU member states (European Commission, 2018), it was reported that most of the systematic improvements in broiler welfare that have occurred since the stocking density standards in the EU broiler directive were implemented result from increased assessment of footpad dermatitis. The emphasis on maintaining good litter quality has also been important, reducing the incidence of coccidiosis and necrotic enteritis and hence the need to use antimicrobials.

One area where high stocking density has been shown to have consistently negative effects is on movement and resting behaviour (see de Jong et al. 2012; Dawkins 2018, for reviews). Even at the highest stocking density allowed in the EU, broilers weighing 3.2 kg have sufficient room to stand and lie down, and in fact occupy only about 77% of the available floor area when doing so (Giersberg et al., 2016). However, multiple studies have also shown that, when broilers are housed at densities above 40 kg/m^2, they jostle one another when moving around, and thus more active birds disturb birds that are trying to rest. In addition, birds are more likely to climb over one another, which can lead to scratches.

Environmental enrichment

There has been increasing interest in providing indoor housed broilers with environmental enrichment, with the goal of stimulating behavioural activity. Broilers in general, and fast-growing broilers in particular, are relatively inactive, particularly as they age. During the first few weeks of life, broilers can regularly be seen to engage in active behaviours like play and walking or running, but older broilers spend most of their time sitting (Bokkers and Koene, 2003; Wallenbeck et al., 2016. It has been suggested that this lack of exercise is a contributing factor to musculoskeletal problems. In addition, providing a more complex and stimulating environment is considered to be beneficial for animal welfare, in that it can promote a wider range of behaviours and allow animals to interact with and explore their environment in a positive way.

A variety of enrichment types have been evaluated for broilers (Figure 3.7). These include structural enrichments (permanent structures added to the house such as perches or platforms), enrichments designed to stimulate foraging behaviour (for example, pecking blocks, feed scattered in the litter), and sensory enrichments (for example, videos, music, odours). Broiler enrichment studies were reviewed recently by Riber et al. (2018). They concluded that the following types showed the most promise for use indoors in commercial facilities, although there were also some potential negative effects.

- **Elevated resting places** (perches and platforms). Chickens are highly motivated to perch in elevated locations, which in the wild serves as an anti-predator behaviour. However, many studies show low use of perches by broilers, probably because perches are not well-designed to support the body size and conformation of commercial broilers. Important factors for heavier birds are also the perch height and ease of accessing the perches (for example, via a ramp rather than having to jump on to the perch). Potential benefits of perches are to improve the ability for birds to thermoregulate

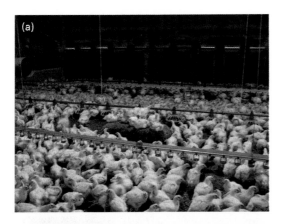

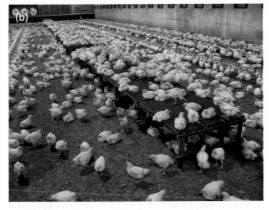

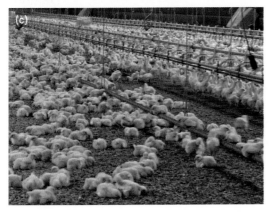

Figure 3.7 Examples of environmental enrichment for broiler chickens: (a) bales; (b) platforms; (c) perches.

under hot conditions because they can get off the litter; reduction in footpad dermatitis; reduction in behavioural disruption; and cleaner plumage. Potential negatives are an increase in breast blisters and keel bone damage (the latter especially in slower-growing birds). No effects of perches on body weight, feed consumption, feed conversion, or fearfulness have been found, and effects on lameness, skeletal disorders and hock burns are inconsistent among studies. Although there are a limited number of studies of platforms (for example, elevated slatted areas above the litter that are accessible via ramps), if well-designed these do appear to be better used by broilers than perches and thus have the potential to improve musculoskeletal condition.

- **Panels/barriers**. Strategically placed panels (or barriers) can visually 'break up' a large house into different sections, and result in more uniform bird distribution, encourage utilisation of under-used areas and reduce behavioural disturbance. They also increase activity since birds have to walk around them. Barriers may directly improve foot and leg health, but this seems to depend upon design factors. However, barriers can impede birds accessing food and water, especially weaker birds.
- **Straw bales**. Bales can act both as barriers and elevated perching surfaces, and can also be used for foraging. Effects on activity and leg problems are inconsistent between studies. Disadvantages are that bales take up a lot of space in the house and can pose biosecurity risks that need to be managed.

Although many third-party animal welfare certification programmes require that broilers be given enrichment, there are still many aspects that require further study. Riber et al. (2018) note that the benefits of particular enrichments should not be generalised, since animal welfare outcomes may depend upon other factors associated with particular housing and management environments, not just enrichment. Further research is needed to refine enrichment design to ensure that the materials used are long lasting and easy to disinfect between flocks. Last, relatively few studies have been carried out in commercial houses, and even fewer have evaluated the optimal placement of enrichments or how many enrichments should be provided in the house to maximise their use and effectiveness in improving broiler welfare. There is also limited information about the on-farm costs associated with implementing enrichment programmes, although in general those studies that have evaluated performance outcomes report little or no negative effects of enrichment provision on growth rates, mortality or feed conversion.

Providing access to the outdoors can also be a form of environmental enrichment, as long as the outdoor area is properly configured and managed to stimulate normal behaviours like foraging while minimising risks of injury, poor ground conditions leading to dirty birds, disease and predation. A major limitation of free-range broiler production is that broilers often either do not leave the house, or if they do leave remain very close to the house after exiting through the pop holes. High bird densities near the pop holes can lead to the ground around the house becoming soiled and denuded.

A variety of factors affect the extent to which broilers use the range. Faster-growing genotypes make less use of the range than slower-growing genotypes (Nielsen et al., 2003; Castellini et al., 2016), and younger broilers range less than older broilers (Stadig et al., 2017). Range use is reduced under poor weather conditions, such as when it is rainy, cold, windy or there is bright sunshine (Dawkins et al., 2003; Stadig et al., 2017; Taylor et al., 2017). Providing either natural or artificial shade/shelter on the range can increase range use and encourage birds to move further from the house (Dawkins et al., 2003; Fanatico et al., 2016; Stadig et al., 2017). Theoretically, the increased activity associated with range use could be beneficial for broiler leg health, but there is limited information on this topic. Several studies have found no or only modest positive effects of range provision on flock leg health (Dawkins et al., 2003; Stadig et al., 2017), whereas others have found more significant effects (Fanatico et al., 2008). Taylor et al. (2018) used a radio frequency identification system to monitor the ranging activity of 538 individual broilers in a commercial flock. They found that the broilers that spent more time on the range had better gait scores, but these broilers also had lower body weights, which could be the major contributor to improved gait.

CHAPTER 4

Health and disease impacts on broiler welfare

CHARLOTTE BERG AND ANDY BUTTERWORTH

The relationship between animal health and animal welfare has been discussed in great detail over the years. Although some people tend to see 'health' as something substantial and measurable, welfare can be perceived as more subjective. We would argue that health is not only the absence of disease and injury, but also references the physical and mental well-being of animals (WHO, 1948; Lerner, 2017), and is an integrated part of the concept of animal welfare. Health problems in broilers leading to clinical symptoms will directly or indirectly affect the welfare of the bird.

In this chapter, we will differentiate between management-related 'disease' and infectious disease.

Such an approach is, of course, partly an illusion, as the risk of infectious diseases is inherently affected by various management decisions

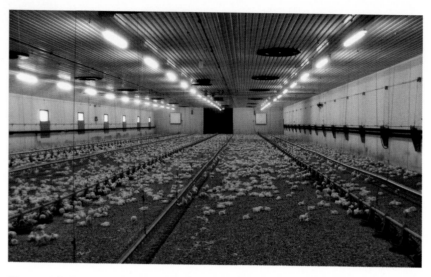

Figure 4.1 To keep the birds healthy, a broiler house needs to provide a suitable environment in terms of temperature, ventilation and litter quality and a high biosecurity level.

and practices at the farm in question. This relates back to the classical concept of the host–agent–environment relationship (Figure 4.1), often described as 'the epidemiologic triangle'. For disease to occur and spread, not only is the presence of a certain microorganism necessary, but there must be a susceptible host (in terms of immune system function, nutritional state, age and other factors). There must also be an environment where the host and the agent meet, directly or via a vector. We can conclude that there is inevitably a management-related factor present in many infectious disease outbreaks. It follows that the difference between infectious and management-related diseases lies mainly in the absence of an infectious agent as the main causative factor in the case of management-related diseases. Nevertheless, the approach of separating the two categories can still be useful for use in the area of broiler health, and we have therefore chosen to retain this separation, after making the readers aware of potential limitations.

During the last decades, the concept of One Health has gained increased popularity among health professionals globally. One Health emphasises the fact that biologically speaking, humans are animals, and that we share, to a substantial extent, our environment and microbes with other domestic or wild animals. This insight is important for combatting severe disease in both humans and domestic animals. Initially, the One Health concept mainly focused on the traditional human medical approach to zoonotic diseases, that is, preventing and controlling a number of diseases in humans by targeting their origins 'at source' – among food producing animals. With time, awareness of the complex pathways of disease or microbe transmission not only from animals to humans but also the other way around, and also of disease transmission between different animal species including vector species, has increased. Furthermore, there is an increasing trend to include not only infectious diseases in the One Health concept (Figure 4.2),

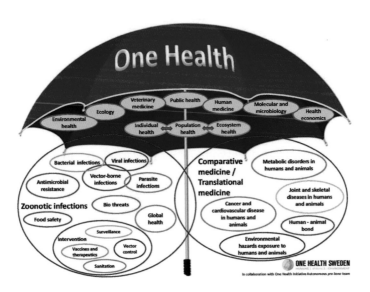

Figure 4.2 The 'One Health Umbrella', illustrating the wide ranging areas brought into the concept.

but also non-infectious diseases, such as metabolic disorders, cancers, cardiovascular disease and environmental hazards. In the following sections, we will focus on the potential welfare consequences for the birds, rather than directly on single named infectious agents, and will also focus on the tools used to diagnose and treat specific conditions – the approach seen in many broiler health textbooks. This is not to, in any way, negate the disease management approach widely used (describe, diagnose, treat) but instead to add a One Health perspective to broiler health discussions. We will also try to relate broiler health to possible consequences for human health and welfare, where this seems possible.

(Partly) management-related diseases

Mortality

Mortality, that is, the proportion of birds dying during rearing from hatching to the pre-slaughter stage at the slaughterhouse, is of course not a disease in itself, but rather a non-specific symptom, and a blunt metric of bird 'health'. Nevertheless, mortality is one of the most widely used, and recorded, measures of broiler health and welfare, and so will not be ignored here.

A dead animal in no longer capable of perceiving anything, including pain or other negative experiences, and so cannot suffer. However, the process of dying, from development of a disease (infectious or not) with potential symptoms including discomfort, pain, distress, frustration and anxiety, to the final collapse of an organ or an organ system, and death, can certainly constitute a welfare problem. This means that the cause of death is a crucial factor when evaluating the relevance of a given mortality level for animal welfare. If death is instantaneous, then no welfare problem exists. However, instantaneous death through disease is not common. If death is slow and painful, and if it involves challenges to bodily functions, and prevents basic behavioural needs from being fulfilled, then the animal welfare consequences can be real and significant. It is generally considered preferable from an animal welfare perspective that as many sick or injured birds as possible are identified and culled at an early stage of the dying process, rather than being left to die on their own (see Chapter 5).

Within commercial broiler production, there are 'expected' (anticipated, and to a degree 'accepted as normal') levels of mortality (Figure 4.3). A certain proportion of the birds 'usually' die during rearing. The actual expected levels will vary depending on genetic hybrid, climate, management system and the age of the bird at slaughter. A rough estimate for a European broiler producer would be that an accumulated broiler mortality of approximately 2–3% for a flock slaughtered at 35–36 days of age is considered 'usual'. As an example, the EU directive regulating

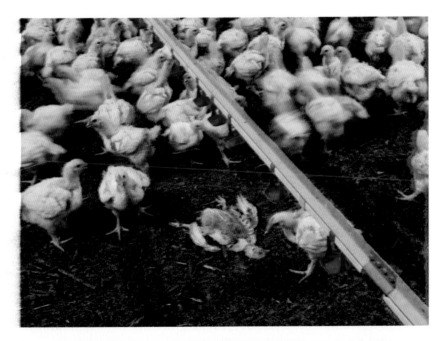

Figure 4.3 A certain level of mortality is anticipated and tolerated within commercial broiler production, but for animal welfare reasons, sick or injured birds should be identified and actively culled rather than left to die in the flock.

the welfare of broilers (Council Directive 2007/43/EC) has a threshold mortality rate of maximum (1% + [0.06% × the age of the flock in days]), averaged over seven consecutive flocks, for producers wanting to apply higher stocking densities. Thus, a broiler flock would be considered to be compliant with the legislation if it had experienced a mortality average of 3.16% at 36 days (average age for seven flocks). Furthermore, several studies have indicated a mortality rate, including culling, of approx. 2.9% for commercial broiler flocks (for example, de Jong et al., 2012).

In large-scale commercial production, individual sick or malformed (for example, birds with severe compromises due to non-infectious skeletal abnormalities) broilers are not treated medically, but are culled. This is because each individual bird has a small economic value, and also to help to prevent disease spread in the flock by rapid removal of compromised individual birds. Keeping broilers in separate sick pens rarely leads to recovery, and retaining sick birds in hospital pens without being able to ensure improvements in their health is not positive for their welfare. Instead, culling is often the recommended option (see Chapter 5).

Skeletal disorders – lameness

Lameness is considered one of the main animal welfare problems within modern broiler production and is one of the major reasons for culling broilers on-farm when this is associated with leg disorders. Broiler lameness is a term which covers a whole range of diseases and skeletal disorders, all resulting in impaired gait, lameness or a complete inability to walk. The causes of broiler lameness may be infectious, in which case they are mainly manifested as joint infection in the hip or tarsal joints; or metabolic, caused by disturbed cartilage or bone development or other deformities occurring as the birds grow. Given the rapid growth of the birds, even a relatively small imbalance of nutrients, nutritional deficiencies, or poor nutrient uptake related to gut health problems can result in significant growth alteration, and so deformities.

The problem of lameness is usually aggravated with increasing age, and potentially as the birds become heavier. However, very lame birds are often small and underweight because mobility compromise has, by then, affected their rate of growth. Higher lameness prevalence is hence more commonly seen in flocks that are reared for slaughter at an older age.

For animal welfare reasons, it is recommended that broilers which show signs of severe lameness are culled. These would include birds which are effectively unable to walk although sometimes move assisted by movement of their wings, or birds which have substantial difficulties in walking, or are unable to stand for a sustained time. Culling is recommended due to the fact that these birds are unlikely to recover (Figure 4.4), and will in some cases be suffering severe pain. Furthermore, birds

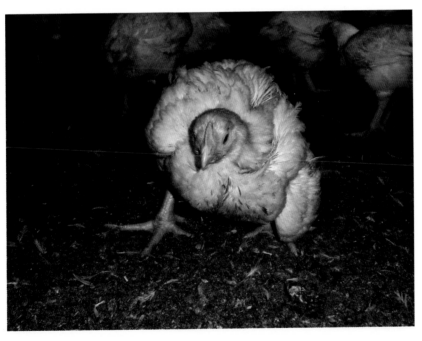

Figure 4.4 For animal welfare reasons, it is recommended that broilers which show signs of severe lameness are culled.

which are unable to walk are often also, as a result of their inability to reach feed and water, suffering from prolonged hunger and thirst, and are often smaller and in poorer body condition than healthy birds in the flock.

Medical or supportive treatment of birds already suffering from severe lameness is normally not an option. However, if a broiler flock is found to have unexpectedly high prevalence of lameness, the cause should be identified in order to take the correct preventive action for consecutive flocks. To achieve this, post-mortem examination of affected birds is recommended. The measures to be taken will be different depending on whether the cause is infectious (for example, femoral head necrosis, infectious synovitis, osteomyelitis), or genetic/nutritional (for example,

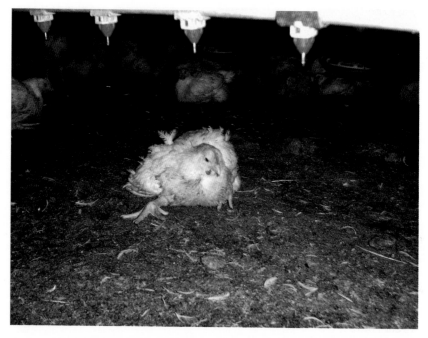

Figure 4.5 Severely lame birds often become underweight, because of their difficulties in reaching feed and water.

tibial dyschondroplasia, angular deformities). As a result of continuous efforts to decrease the incidence of hereditary disease on broiler lameness, the incidence of leg problems has decreased over the last decades. However, in some countries – due to nutritional and disease challenge effects – lameness remains a significant cause of production losses and poor bird welfare. The gait abnormalities seen in birds with medium gait compromise (up to gait score 3, Kestin et al., 1992) are not necessarily linked to obvious post-mortem pathological findings but may be related to the general body shape of the broiler, which is influenced by the high relative mass of breast muscle. However, very lame birds (gait score 4 and 5, Kestin et al., 1992) are usually small and underweight for their age (Figure 4.5), as they have been compromised in their capacity to access resources including food and water. This point is often not understood, and many commentators state (wrongly) that broiler lameness is due to body conformation in heavy weight birds, which is absolutely not the case for very lame birds – which struggle to reach water drinkers and cannot move between feed pans and drinkers.

Contact dermatitis

Contact dermatitis (Figure 4.6) is a term usually used to describe a range of pathologies affecting the skin of broilers. It is usually related to contact with wet or dirty litter, and mainly affects the footpads, hocks and, in severe cases, also the breast region. The condition(s) are sometimes referred to as footpad dermatitis, pododermatitis, hock burn and breast blisters, respectively (Berg, 2004).

Skin lesions can be seen, perhaps surprisingly, when the birds are less than 1 week old. However, they are usually more prevalent as the birds become older, as litter quality deteriorates and the birds spend more time sitting down and hence more time with their hocks and breast in direct contact with the litter. Litter moisture is the main factor affecting the incidence of the problem. Litter quality and friability can in turn be influenced by factors such as feed composition, gut health, leaks and

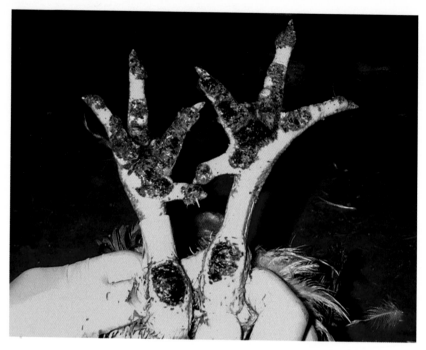

Figure 4.6 A case of severe footpad dermatitis and hock burn in a 35-day-old broiler. The ulcers are covered by dark crusts, to which litter and faecal material has adhered.

poor maintenance of the water distribution system, stocking density, season, ventilation capacity and air humidity (Ekstrand et al., 1998; de Jong et al., 2012).

Contact dermatitis is manifested as dark lesions, where the normal skin pattern is disrupted. In mild cases, hyperkeratosis and discoloration is seen. If aggravated, superficial skin lesions can progress further into ulcers, causing pain and swelling. In the case of footpad dermatitis, usually both feet are affected, and birds may not appear lame, but may walk with a hobbling gait (as both feet are symmetrically affected). The severe lesions are considered painful (Berg, 2004). It has been shown that birds with severe footpad dermatitis (often referred to as FPD) grow more slowly, and hence there are economic incentives, in addition to the animal welfare reasons, for trying to reduce the prevalence of the disease.

In general, mild contact dermatitis may not have negative effects on the welfare of individual birds. However, at the flock level a high incidence of mild dermatitis can be an indicator of overall problems in the house environment with respect to wet litter, which can in turn be linked to inadequate ventilation, poorly designed, adjusted or maintained water supply equipment, overstocking, dietary imbalances, gut infections, and also to other management-related factors. Contact dermatitis can be, and is, thus used as a more generalised broiler welfare indicator. Presence of footpad dermatitis not only constitutes a possible bird welfare problem itself (at least if the lesions are severe) but can also reflect the presence of other risk factors for impaired welfare related to air quality, litter quality, space allowance and so on.

Metabolic disorders

The relatively rapid growth of the modern broiler involves a certain risk of metabolic disorders. The two main ones are ascites and sudden death syndrome (SDS).

Ascites (Figure 4.7) is caused by tissue fluid accumulating inside the bird's abdomen, compromising body shape, and is related to the bird's cardiovascular function (Olkowski et al., 2005). The bird walks with a strange body posture and its growth rate is affected. Ascites usually progresses slowly, with the abdomen gradually becoming extended and the centre of gravity of the bird being gradually shifted. The fluid accumulation will, in addition, affect organ function. Given the chronic nature of the condition, ascites constitutes a considerable bird welfare problem for affected individuals.

SDS, on the other hand, usually affects big, heavy birds that have been performing well in terms of growth, and then suddenly 'flip over' (the

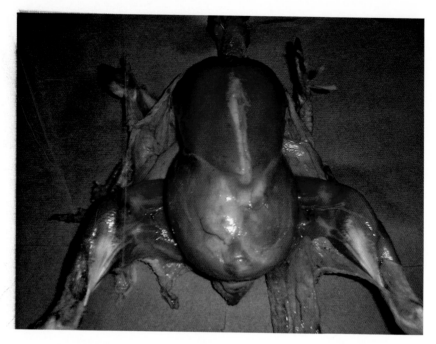

Figure 4.7 Broiler with the distended and fluid filled abdomen seen in ascites. Photo: Andy Grist.

condition is hence sometimes referred to as 'flip over' by producers) and die. The condition is believed to be related to a malfunction in the heart. There are no pre-indications that the birds are experiencing poor welfare prior to their sudden death, and due to its acute nature (the bird dies rather rapidly), the condition is not considered to be of major animal welfare importance. Nevertheless, sudden death inevitably limits longevity and mainly affects birds approaching the planned slaughter age, and so is of production relevance.

Respiratory and mucous membrane problems

Broilers reared in houses with poor air quality, especially in relation to dust and high ammonia concentrations, may suffer from the direct effects of pollutants on mucous membranes and through damage to their respiratory organs. There may also be indirect effects, as poor air quality may be detrimental to the general disease resistance of the birds. This is all linked to the broiler house environment and can, for example, result from poorly designed, maintained, or managed ventilation, unsuitable litter material, dusty feed or overcrowding, causing poor litter conditions. Often respiratory disease problems will not be cured by medication alone, but by better management, at least for the next flocks of birds.

Physical injuries

Injuries to individual birds in poultry flocks can occur if birds come into contact with poorly designed or maintained house features, or via interactions with other birds in the flock. Modern broiler houses are designed to be relatively easy to clean, which is beneficial to both the producer and the birds. Nevertheless, equipment will be present, such as feeder and drinker lines, feed hoppers, heating equipment (brooders, space heaters, heat exchangers), step on weighing scales (in some farms), and equipment for collecting dead birds. Although accidents are rare, they can happen, and it is the responsibility of producer to ensure that birds are not injured by sharp protruding objects, caught in wires or otherwise injure themselves unnecessarily. Broiler are generally not prone to hysteria or smothering, but producers should nevertheless take care to ensure that people who move within a flock do so gently and calmly, to avoid causing panic or accidentally stepping on birds that are not moving away rapidly enough.

Broilers are immature animals. They are usually slaughtered when they are not yet adults – and at that age they have little tendency towards aggression or feather pecking. It is usually possible to apply reasonably high levels of illumination without triggering injurious pecking in these birds, and in some countries broilers are routinely reared in almost daylight (Figure 4.8) levels as the sides of the houses are made of mesh open to bright daylight.

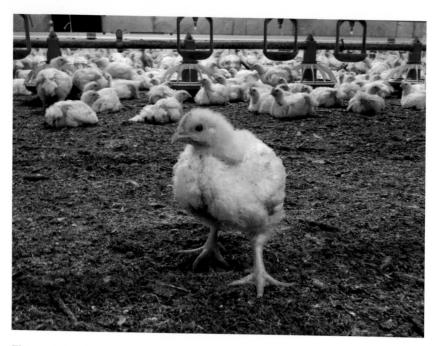

Figure 4.8 It is usually possible to apply reasonably high light levels without triggering any tendencies of injurious pecking in broilers.

Peritonitis and septicaemia

Peritonitis, endocarditis and septicaemia are rather common causes of mortality in broilers (Kittelsen et al., 2015). While these diseases are all related to microbial pathogens, they do not typically spread to a large number of birds, that is, these diseases do not show the 'contagious disease' pattern. Instead, single birds are affected, in what can be described as an erratic pattern, quite unpredictable and scattered. Affected birds will usually deteriorate rapidly, and should be culled to prevent further suffering, and potentially to reduce the risk of spread to other birds in close proximity. It is difficult to identify a clear cause of the diseases, and although a post-mortem examination will often reveal the presence of *E. coli* bacteria, such bacteria are also present in many healthy

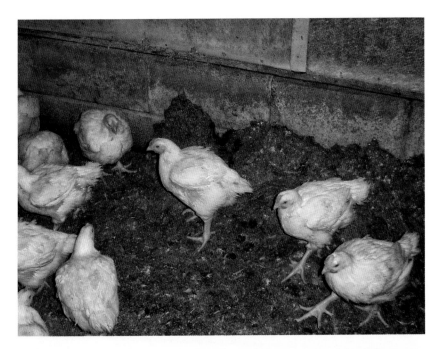

Figure 4.9 Poor cleaning in between flocks increases the risk of disease in the birds. In old buildings with cracked floors, non-smooth walls and wooden constructions, cleaning and disinfection between consecutive flocks can be quite difficult.

birds. Good hygiene procedures, especially in relation to cleaning and disinfection (Figure 4.9) between consecutive flocks, is usually the main recommendation in relation to this problem.

Runting

Single birds which are not growing in accordance with to the expected rate are known as runts, and these birds fall behind their flock mates in terms of size and feather development. Such birds do not necessarily look or behave as if they are sick. On the contrary, they may be quite active, running around more than their heavier flock mates are, and appear healthy. It cannot be said that runting birds are necessarily suffering, and a post-mortem examination will not necessarily reveal any clear cause of the impaired growth rate and late development. However, there are still animal welfare risks related to runts, the main one being poor access to water, as the producer will gradually elevate the drinker (and feeder) lines as the main proportion of the flock grows, eventually making it impossible for the runts to reach these resources. Therefore, the recommendation is to cull runts (Figure 4.10) before they fall too much behind. Furthermore, experience shows that runts very rarely catch up with their flock mates with time, which means that at the day of slaughter they will still be much smaller than the other birds in the flock. Once at the slaughterhouse, they will cause disruption to the process or – worst case – in the case of electrical waterbath stunners, be too

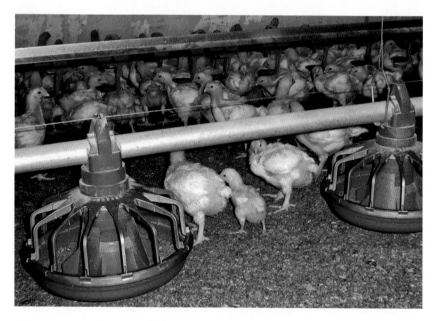

Figure 4.10 Runts may appear healthy but there are still animal welfare risks related to not culling these birds, as they may experience poor access to water as the producer gradually elevates the drinker lines as the flock grows.

small for the shackles or too short to reach the stunning waterbath, and hence risk being bled without prior stunning, which is not acceptable. For the combination of these reasons, runts should be culled on-farm, preferably when first detected, and must be culled prior to transport to protect them from the risk of not being effectively stunned.

Other non-contagious diseases and conditions

This chapter does not cover a complete or exhaustive list of management and housing-related health and welfare problems in broilers. Additionally, there are health problems that may be of regional importance, but only in a limited geographical area, and these are not mentioned here.

One problem attracting increasing attention during the last decade or so is myopathies (myo = muscle, pathy = pathology of; myopathy = localised disorder of muscle), such as wooden-breast, white striping or so-called 'spaghetti meat' in broiler breast fillets. These abnormalities certainly constitute a product quality issue, and are believed to be linked to the genetic selection for muscle hypertrophy (rapid growth of muscle) in fast-growing broiler strains, combined with nutritional factors – perhaps insufficiency of some specific nutrients to supply rapid muscle fibre growth, leading to locally insufficient blood supply and muscle hypoxia (Petracci et al., 2019). There are animal welfare concerns in relation to these conditions, as the localised tissues, particularly in the breast muscles, may become inflamed or necrotic. However, from an action point of view, the key to these problems appears to lie in the hands of the geneticists, and perhaps in poultry nutritionists, and not, in general, with the individual farmer or veterinarian.

Infectious diseases

Existing textbooks on broiler welfare often do not focus much on infectious and contagious disease. However, it is important to keep in mind that infections and disease can certainly result in considerable bird welfare problems linked to the symptoms of the disease, morbidity, depression, immobility, 'sickness behaviours', inappetence, weight loss and mortality after prolonged suffering in the case where the sick bird is not detected and treated, or culled. Additionally, procedures related to on-farm killing of affected flocks can have significant welfare implications – for example, how does one kill 150,000 broilers, on a farm, in a controlled and humane manner in the face of a disease outbreak?

The key to avoid broilers being affected by contagious diseases is, of course, good biosecurity and proper health management plans, including use of effectively managed vaccination. In general, birds enter the farm as single-age groups in many farms (but in some very large farms, the birds are of different ages in different houses). The rather simple and barren layout of broiler sheds in temperate climates is an advantage from a biosecurity point of view, as the surfaces and equipment are easier to clean between flocks. Birds reared indoors in climate-controlled houses should have no contact with wild birds or rodents, and any visitors entering the facilities should be expected to change clothes and boots, and wash their hands prior to contact with any live birds. Most often, there are no enrichment objects, and although this may be negative from a bird activity and movement perspective, it also means a low risk of introducing pathogens through objects in the house. The balance between enrichment and hygienic blandness may suggest that enrichments are a hazard, but they do not need to be – it is relatively easy to provide cleanable enrichments (platforms, pecking objects, bales of new litter material) without damaging the biosecurity protection for the birds.

The use of vaccines for broilers differs substantially between countries and regions, as a result of differences in management practices, disease prevalence and national policies. In many countries, parent stock are vaccinated against a considerable range of diseases, and the immunity transferred to the embryos is then sometimes considered sufficient for the broilers during production. In consequence no, or few, vaccinations are then used on the offspring chicks. To determine what, and if, any vaccinations are necessary, it is crucial to be well informed about the disease and vaccination status of the parent stock and other poultry in the region. Furthermore, vaccine availability and also legal restrictions may differ between regions.

Diseases of relevance

Some diseases of broilers can be considered endemic, that is, the pathogen is present in some poultry flocks and/or in other species in the region. Examples of such diseases include the parasitic coccidiosis (Figure 4.11) (virtually all conventionally reared broiler flocks routinely receive feed containing anti-coccidial drugs during the rearing period except for a number of days prior to slaughter, that is, the withdrawal time), and bacterial diseases such as those caused by *Campylobacter*

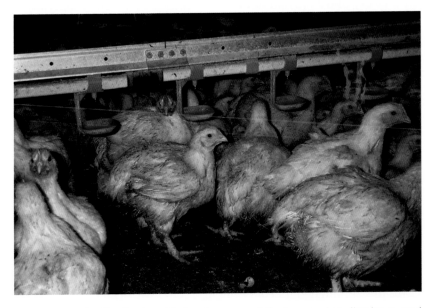

Figure 4.11 Broiler flock suffering from coccidiosis, causing diarrhoea and soiled plumage.

spp., and in some regions also at least some strains of *Salmonella* spp. Some viral diseases, including Marek's disease (caused by an avian alphaherpesvirus), Gumboro disease (infectious bursitis, caused by a birnavirus, infectious bursal disease virus) may cause disease symptoms by themselves but also have a general immunosuppressive effect, thereby making the birds more sensitive to other, usually secondary bacterial, infections as well. It should be stressed that the fact that a disease is considered endemic does not mean that it is acceptable for all flocks to be infected by these pathogenic agents. Good biosecurity routines can still make a large difference in protecting birds from disease, and hence help to protect their welfare.

Then there are other diseases which are commonly referred to as 'exotic', that is, non-endemic. However, one should bear in mind that a disease that is endemic in one country, could be regarded as exotic in another. Examples of such diseases are Newcastle disease (caused by avian paramyxovirus), and AI (avian influenza) (caused by a range of subtypes of avian influenza virus), where, when the disease is detected, an elimination procedure will be considered, that is, killing of all infected flocks and possibly also in contact flocks (flocks in close proximity). Outbreaks of such disease can have severe broiler welfare consequences. First, the affected birds will become ill and may suffer before they die from the disease. Second, the on-farm killing methods can involve procedures that are far from ideal from a bird welfare point of view. To prevent unplanned reaction to these kinds of emergency situations, national contingency plans should be in place, indicating what methods will be used in the case of depopulation for disease control purposes (Figure 4.12) and how animal welfare risks will be minimised (Berg, 2012). This involves proper monitoring of bird welfare during the entire process.

Furthermore, outbreaks of exotic disease can lead to other measures being imposed by the authorities on broiler farms and other poultry farms in a certain region. For example, a stand-still of all poultry-related transports might be imposed, rapidly leading to welfare problems on some farms. These can occur through overcrowding as the birds continue

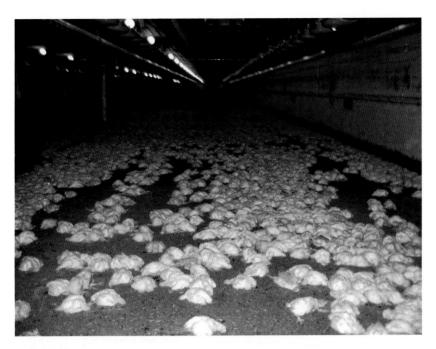

Figure 4.12 Killing of broilers for disease control purposes, using carbon dioxide, whole-house gassing. Photo courtesy: J. Wehre.

to grow while not being allowed to be sent for slaughter (Figure 4.13), and slaughterhouses might also be shut-down to prevent further spread of the disease. In these cases, emergency depopulation may be the only remaining option, although the farms themselves are not infected.

Finally, it should be borne in mind that there are diseases that are not primarily harmful to the broilers themselves, but which may still be problematic in relation to human health, as they are zoonotic. Examples are *Campylobacter* spp. infections or some species of *Salmonella*, which will not cause clinical disease in the birds but may nevertheless pose a threat to human health. In these cases, the One Health perspective is highly relevant, as it incorporates processes aimed at minimising infection transfer from, for example, broilers to humans. Hence, depopulation may, for example, be the decision chosen for a broiler flock infected with *Salmonella*, even though the specific serotype does not cause disease in the birds.

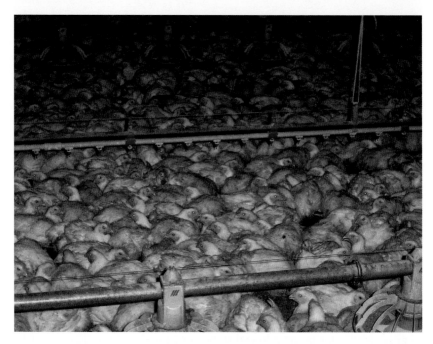

Figure 4.13 Disease outbreaks in a region may lead to involuntary overstocking, including at non-infected farms, if birds cannot be transported to the slaughterhouse as planned.

CHAPTER 5

On-farm and casualty slaughter welfare of broilers

MOHAN RAJ AND CHARLOTTE BERG

Broiler production involves rearing of both sexes for meat. A small proportion of newly hatched chicks that are considered to be unviable or deformed, and embryos (unhatched or 'pipped' eggs) are routinely killed in hatcheries. The numbers of these killed in hatcheries vary according to the size of the operation and efficacy of the incubation systems (setters and hatchers), in particular, temperature, humidity and gas levels. Efficient control of these variables is vital to minimising loss.

The producer and stockpersons at a broiler farm are responsible for ensuring that birds that are suffering from injury or disease, where treatment is not an option (for practical, medical or financial reasons), are humanely killed. According to the EU broiler directive (Council Directive 2007/43/EC), broiler keepers are obliged to participate in specific training, including emergency killing and culling. Furthermore, the owner or keeper shall provide instructions and guidance concerning the methods of culling birds practised in the holding, to other persons employed or otherwise engaged there.

In general broilers achieve the target market size in around 5 to 6 weeks with a live weight of 2–2.5 kg. The live weights farmers produce depend on the market in a specific country, region or the market segment that has to be supplied. The vast majority of broilers are kept in large groups in closed, controlled housing systems. It is known that health and survival of broiler chicks during the first week of life depend on the genetic line of the breeders, breeder age, egg weight, egg storage conditions and duration, and incubation conditions and altitude. In commercial broiler flocks single birds are rarely treated or placed in separate sick pens. Instead, birds that are not fit to follow the routines in the large flocks are normally removed and destroyed. Also, birds that are not apparently sick but who are growing considerably slower than the remaining flock, so-called 'runts', will usually be culled. The reason for this is twofold: first, as feed and water lines are gradually elevated to fit the size of the birds, the runts may experience difficulties reaching these resources and consequently suffer from prolonged thirst and hunger. Second, these very small birds are usually not accepted by the slaughterhouse, even if they survived the last journey, as they do not fit the stunning and processing equipment. The EU Regulation 1099/2009 clearly states that birds that are likely to miss the water bath stunners, which is the most common method used throughout the world, should not be shackled, but instead killed humanely. Furthermore, birds that are not fit for transport should not be transported, but instead killed humanely on the farm to avoid unnecessary suffering during transport.

Hence broiler chickens may have to be killed on the farm during production for health, welfare or economic reasons. For example, newly hatched chicks derive nutrients from their yolk sacks for survival for the first few days of life (up to 72 hours after hatching) and may not survive if they do not begin to eat and drink before this source is depleted.

Broiler farmers therefore routinely monitor the flock and they recognise chicks' viability from their growth and activity patterns. Inevitably, chicks showing signs of poor health and viability will have to be killed, which is commonly known as 'culling', and is a continuous operation throughout the production cycle in broiler flock. Culling is economically advantageous because it helps to save feed costs by the avoidance of feeding birds that would not reach slaughter weight anyway, prevent the spread of diseases and achieve uniformity of the flock weight.

Another major reason for culling broilers on-farm is associated with leg disorders (see Chapter 4). Infectious causes of leg disorders may begin in the flock as early as 14 days of age and worsen very rapidly during 25 to 45 days of age. It is a common practice in the industry to cull broilers showing signs of severe lameness, that is, birds being unable to walk or having great difficulties in walking or sustained standing, due to the fact that these birds will in many cases be suffering severe pain and they would, as a result of their increasing immobility, be deprived of access to feed and water. The prevalence of severe leg weakness, as in severely affected mobility, in commercial broiler flocks has been estimated to be up to 5–6% in various older scientific studies (Kestin et al., 1992; Sanotra et al., 2003). Considerable breeding efforts have been made to decrease the magnitude of the problem over the last decades, and it has been shown that the gait abnormalities seen nowadays are not necessarily linked to obvious post-mortem pathological findings (Sandilands et al., 2011; de Jong et al., 2012). Nevertheless, severely impaired gait should still be a reason for culling, regardless of the underlying cause. Other reasons for culling include ascites, injuries and unspecific signs of disease, such as dullness and apathy.

Good farming practice should include keeping of verifiable records concerning the number of birds, reasons and method used for culling of broilers. Records showing the number of broilers found dead and an indication of the causes, and the number of birds culled with cause, is a requirement stated in the EU broiler directive (Council Directive 2007/43/EC). Furthermore, if producers want to apply the higher stocking densities in accordance with the directive, an upper limit with respect to the cumulative daily mortality is set to 1% + 0.06% multiplied by the slaughter age of the flock in days, to be applied on a number of consecutive flocks from a house. This means that for a broiler flock slaughtered at 35 days of age a mortality of no more than 3.1% is considered acceptable by the industry on economic grounds, including both birds found dead and birds having been culled. Studies from several European countries have indicated a mortality rate, including culling, of approximately 2.9% for commercial broiler flocks with fast-growing strains (de Jong et al., 2011a, 2011b).

In general, it is considered preferable from an animal welfare perspective that as many sick or injured birds as possible are identified and culled at an early stage, rather than left to die on their own. This is of course related to the cause of mortality and the process of dying, prior to the instance of death. The exact instance of death is not considered painful in itself, but the time prior to death may involve severe suffering. Some health problems may lead to apparent sudden death without prior symptoms in the birds, but in many cases there will be a period of deteriorated health prior to death. A bird that is suffering from a disease, experiencing pain, fatigue and severe physical and mental stress during a long period of time from first developing signs of disease, ending up being unable to move, possibly permanently recumbent, until finally succumbing to death, will experience more suffering than a bird being euthanised when first showing signs of incurable disease. Hence, the ratio of culled birds versus total mortality can be considered an animal welfare indicator. If the producer/stockperson is skilled and rigorous when inspecting the flock on a daily basis, the chances of detecting birds that should be culled increases, and fewer birds are left to die slowly and painfully.

The impact of disease on welfare of broilers has been addressed previously (Butterworth and Weeks, 2010). Stunning and slaughter in slaughterhouses for human consumption and depopulation have been covered in the previous publication (Gerritzen and Gibson, 2016; Raj and

Velarde, 2016; Velarde and Raj, 2016). Therefore, scope of this chapter will be restricted to methods that could be used for emergency killing of broilers and killing of unwanted chicks and embryos in hatcheries. Some of these methods could also be used for on-farm killing of broilers for human consumption.

Legal framework and guidelines

There are several terminologies representing circumstances under which broilers may have to be killed on-farm. For example, the European slaughter and killing regulation (Council Regulation 1099/2009) provides the following definitions:

- killing means any intentionally induced process which causes the death of an animal
- emergency killing means the killing of animals which are injured or have a disease associated with severe pain or suffering and where there is no other practical possibility to alleviate this pain or suffering
- stunning means any intentionally induced process which causes loss of consciousness and sensibility without pain, including any process resulting in instantaneous death
- slaughtering means the killing of animals intended for human consumption
- depopulation means the process of killing animals for public health, animal health, animal welfare or environmental reasons under the supervision of the competent authority.

In this regulation, *simple stunning* refers to reversible loss of consciousness and *stunning* refers to irreversible loss of consciousness in animals.

There are also several international institutional guidelines for killing animals, including broilers, on-farm available for consultation.

American Veterinary Medical Association (AVMA):

- https://www.avma.org/KB/Policies/Pages/Euthanasia-Guidelines.aspx
- https://www.avma.org/KB/Resources/Reference/AnimalWelfare/Pages/Depopulation.aspx

European Food Safety Authority (EFSA):

- http://onlinelibrary.wiley.com/doi/10.2903/j.efsa.2004.45/pdf

World Organisation for Animal Health (OIE):

- http://www.oie.int/eng/normes/mcode/en_chapitre_3.7.6.htm

Humane Slaughter Association:

- https://www.hsa.org.uk/downloads/technical-notes/TN11-on-farm-poultry-large-flock-slaughter.pdf
- https://www.hsa.org.uk/downloads/publications/hsa-practical-slaughter-of-poultry.pdf

EU Commission:

- https://eur-lex.europa.eu/legal-content/EN/TXT/PDF/?uri=CELEX:32009R1099&from=EN
- https://ec.europa.eu/food/sites/food/files/animals/docs/aw_prac_slaughter_factsheet-2018_handle_poultry_en.pdf
- https://ec.europa.eu/food/sites/food/files/animals/docs/aw_prac_slaughter_factsheet-2018_stun_poultry_en.pdf
- https://ec.europa.eu/food/sites/food/files/animals/docs/aw_prac_slaughter_factsheet-2018_farm_poultry_en.pdf

The EU Regulation 1099/2009 lists stunning or killing methods that could be used under different circumstances.

1. Mechanical methods:

- penetrative captive bolt
- non-penetrative captive bolt
- firearm with free projectile
- maceration (chicks up to 72 hours)
- manual or mechanical cervical dislocation (up to 3 kg live weight for manual and up to 5 kg live weight for mechanical)
- percussive blow to the head (up to 5 kg live weight).

2. Electrical methods:

- head-only electrical stunning
- head-to-body electrical stunning
- electrical waterbath.

3. Gaseous methods:

- carbon dioxide at high concentrations ($>40\%$)
- carbon dioxide in two phases
- carbon dioxide associated with inert gases
- inert gases
- carbon monoxide ($>4\%$) (can be used when carcasses are not intended for human consumption)
- carbon monoxide associated with other gases ($>1\%$) (can be used when carcasses are not intended for human consumption)

Gases can be administered in containers or to previously sealed houses (that is, whole-house gassing and removal of dead birds). Other methods include lethal injection, which can be used when carcasses are not intended for human consumption.

It should be mentioned that individual EU member states may have chosen to adopt stricter national legislation regarding which of the above-mentioned methods to allow and how various methods are to be applied. It is the responsibility of the person who is trained in carrying out broiler killing or culling to ensure that international and national legislation is complied with. Application of a simple stunning method should be followed by a killing procedure and death should be confirmed before carcass disposal or processing.

Killing of chicks and embryos in hatcheries

The EU regulation (Council Regulation 1099/2009) stipulates that the maceration method, when used, should provide instantaneous maceration and immediate death of the chicks and embryos. The apparatus should contain rapidly rotating mechanically operated killing blades or expanded polystyrene projections. The capacity of the apparatus shall be sufficient to ensure that all chicks are killed instantaneously, even if they are handled in a large number. It should be emphasised that the equipment does not primarily operate by cutting the chicks, which means that the sharpness of the blades is not crucial. In any event, mechanical destruction of chicks should result in slurry, rather than recognisable body parts such as internal organs, legs, wings and heads, to ensure chicks were truly macerated. Garden shredders should not be used.

As a guide to good practice, the mechanically operated rotating blades should be rotating at a speed of at least 2000 revolutions per minute (RPM). The gap between expanded polystyrene projections should be set as narrow as possible to ensure chicks' heads are crushed instantaneously leading to death. If the gap is wide (for example, more than 10 mm), the chicks' abdomens will be crushed without causing any damage to the brain required to attain unconsciousness, leading to serious welfare compromise.

In some hatcheries, chicks are separated from embryos and killed by manual cervical dislocation (small hatcheries) or exposed to gas mixtures, usually carbon dioxide, whereas the embryos are conveyed into a macerator.

On-farm killing of broilers

Captive bolts

Penetrative and non-penetrative captive bolts (Figure 5.1) have been developed owing to the welfare concern that cervical dislocation does not necessarily cause brain concussion in poultry. These captive bolt guns could be powered by using either cartridges or compressed air (Raj and O'Callaghan, 2001; see also https://www.acclesandshelvoke.co.uk/media/downloads/2017/August/data-sheets/CASH-Small-Animal-Tool-JUN-2017.pdf). The key captive bolt parameters are bolt diameter, velocity and penetration depth. In this regard, the ideal variables for stunning/killing broilers with a captive bolt are reported to be a minimum of 6 mm diameter driven perpendicular to the skull with an airline pressure of 827 kPa and a penetration depth of 10 mm (Raj and O'Callaghan, 2001). Birds can be restrained manually or in a cone or shackle for the purpose of application. When the muzzle of the gun is placed on the head and fired, the impact of the bolt on the skull produces fractures and severe brain injury, leading to death (Figure 5.1). Some retailers' in the UK recommend these guns as preferred killing method for broilers. In some countries, the captive bolt shot is only considered a stunning method, and death then has to be ensured by bleeding or neck dislocation. Also spring-operated captive bolt guns are available on the market (see, for example, Sparrey et al., 2014). Anecdotal evidence, however, suggests that the spring-operated

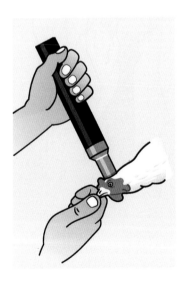

Figure 5.1 Illustration of captive bolt stunning. Source: Factsheet published by the European Commission.

captive bolt guns are usually not powerful enough to ensure efficient stunning.

Captive bolt stunning of broilers of all ages leads to severe wing flapping due to the destruction of the brain and spillage of brain particles and blood through the fractured skull. Therefore, it would be better to perform stunning outside the growing shed and place the captive bolt-stunned poultry in a bin to collect spillage, for biosecurity reasons. Death can be confirmed after the cessation of wing flapping, and dilated pupils and absence of breathing can be used as indicators of death.

Cervical dislocation

Manual cervical dislocation (Figure 5.2) is frequently used on farms to dispose small broilers (less than 3 kg live weight). Broiler breeders (up to 5 kg), however, would require mechanical devices to perform cervical dislocation. Research has shown that dislocation caused by neck stretching is more humane than that caused by neck crushing (see, for example, Sparrey et al., 2014), the latter does not always induce signs of brain concussion. For cervical dislocation to be humane, it should be performed in one stretch and result in severance of spinal cord from the brain and cessation of blood supply to the brain via severance of both carotid arteries. In some countries, a separate stunning method, such as a percussive blow to the head, is required for broilers (except for small chicks) prior to killing by neck

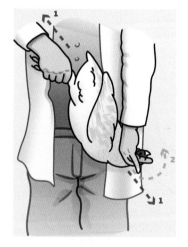

Figure 5.2 Illustration of and instruction for cervical dislocation. Source: Factsheet published by the European Commission.

In one continuous movement:

1. Pull both hands **quickly and firmly** in opposite directions
2. Snap the head back sharply

dislocation, to ensure that birds are unconscious before neck dislocation attempts are carried out.

Cervical dislocation also leads to severe wing flapping due to separation of spinal cord from the brain, which is mandatory, and frequently leads to decapitation. Cervical dislocated broilers can be placed in a bin to avoid spillage of blood and death confirmed after the cessation of wing flapping. Dilated pupils and absence of breathing can be used as indicators of death.

Blow to the head

Percussive blow to the head can be delivered using a blunt object (for example, baton or club) and a single blow should render the bird unconscious and both carotid arteries must be severed immediately to ensure death. A percussive blow to the head can also be achieved by holding the bird's body by both hands and rapidly swinging it in such a way that the bird's head hits a hard, stationary object, such as the rim of a table. However, the operators' competency and compassion are key to achieving effective stunning/killing. Cessation of bleeding through the neck cut wound, dilated pupils and absence of breathing can be used as indicators of death.

Head-only electrical stunning

Head-only electrical stunning followed by severance of both carotid arteries is normally used when broilers are slaughtered on-farm for human consumption. The stunning electrodes are placed on either side of the head (Figure 5.3) of a bird restrained in a cone or shackle, and a minimum current of 240 mA (according to the EU Regulation) applied for at least 7 seconds to induce a generalised epileptiform activity in the brain, indicative of unconsciousness. Both carotid arteries should be cut as soon as possible, to ensure rapid onset of death. Research has shown that electrical waveform, voltage and minimum current

Figure 5.3 Head-only electrical stunning tong position. Source: Factsheet published by the European Commission.

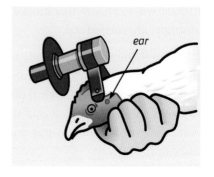

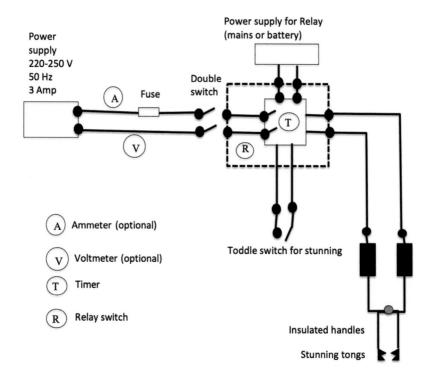

Step-up transformer will be necessary where the mains supply voltage is 110V.

Figure 5.4 Schematic diagram for a head-only electrical stunner for poultry.

delivered to birds are key parameters that determine the induction and maintenance of unconsciousness until death occurs through blood loss (Raj and O'Callaghan, 2004). Electrical stunners can be constructed using the scheme presented in the Figure 5.4. Such head-only stunning equipment, followed by neck dislocation or bleeding, can of course also be used for killing broilers in other situations than slaughter for human consumption. It should, however, be emphasised that in the case of killing for disease control purposes, it is often preferred, for biosecurity reasons, to apply methods not involving bleeding, to minimise contamination.

Head-only electrical stunning tongs should be cleaned prior to use, for example, by using a wire brush, as dirt and feather accumulating in the tongs would not only increase electrical resistance leading to localised heating effect causing carbonisation, but also electrical arc, reducing the efficacy of stunning. Electrical stunning current of at least 240 mA should be applied uninterruptedly for at least 4 seconds. Health and safety of operators should be paramount while using hand-held electrical stunning devices, especially during wing flapping that occurs during and after stunning. Therefore, standard operating procedure should include provision of all the necessary personnel protection equipment.

Head-only electrical stunning leads to severe wing flapping from the moment stunning current is switched on, which would interfere with prompt and accurate neck cutting. Owing to this, broilers should be ideally restrained in a cone prior to stunning or placed in a cone immediately after stunning and both the carotid arteries supplying oxygenated blood to the brain must be severed as soon as possible, in any case no later than 15 seconds. Wing flapping occurs as a part of the generalised epileptiform activity in the brain, induced by the stunning current, and it could last for several seconds. EU Regulation 1099/2009 stipulates that carcass processing can only begin after confirmation of death in animals, including poultry. Cessation of bleeding through the neck cut wound, dilated pupils and absence of breathing can be used as indicators of death.

Head-to-body electrical stunning

Head-to-body electrical stunning is not used in poultry although exper-imental prototype equipment has been developed and tested (Raj et al., 2001). Broilers may be killed if the method induces cardiac arrest and therefore neck cutting may not be necessary where carcasses are not intended for human consumption. Dilated pupils and absence of breathing can be used as indicators of death.

Waterbath stunning

Although uncommon, electrical waterbath stunning can be used to stun broilers on farms, and the minimum currents prescribed in EU Regulation 1099/2009 are listed in Table 5.1. The minimum current should be applied for at least four seconds. Both carotid arteries must be severed as soon as possible when *simple stunning* is used, that is, when cardiac arrest is not induced at water bath stunning.

Effective electrical water bath stunning leads to a state of tetanus, known as tonic seizure, lasting several seconds, during which the wings are held tightly around the breast, legs are extended and neck arched. Muscular tremors may also occur. Effective neck cutting of broilers during the epileptic state leads to rapid onset of death in unconscious broilers. Cessation of bleeding through the neck cut wound, dilated pupils and absence of breathing can be used as indicators of death.

Table 5.1 Waterbath stunning minimum currents (EU Regulation 1099/2009).

Frequency (Hz)	Current per bird (mA)
< 200	100
200–400	150
400–1500	200

Gas mixtures

Most gaseous methods are mainly used in slaughterhouse settings or at hatcheries, as they can be rather complicated. However, in situations where entire flocks of broilers are to be killed, for disease control purposes or for animal welfare reasons (in case of severe neglect, or when a disease outbreak prevents the transportation of feed to the farm or of birds to the slaughterhouse), such methods may nevertheless be relevant. The same applies to the killing of batches of broilers involved in severe traffic accidents, where further transportation is not considered feasible or acceptable from an animal welfare point of view.

In these cases, the methods mentioned above for culling small numbers of birds may not be practically feasible, given the number of broilers involved in cases of total depopulation. Instead, gaseous methods are then usually applied. These include either bringing the birds to a container unit where carbon dioxide at high concentrations or inert gases are used, or applying whole-house gas killing with carbon dioxide at high concentrations. Killing on-farm at depopulation has been covered in the previous publication (Gerritzen and Gibson, 2016) and will hence not be described in further detail here.

Nevertheless, individual or small groups of birds could be placed in an open-top box into which a gas that is heavier than air, such as argon or carbon dioxide, can be slowly filled with increasing concentrations leading to lethal level achieved. While using argon, the residual oxygen level should be reduced to below 2% by volume; while using carbon dioxide, a minimum of 45% by volume should be attained. Broilers require 2 minutes exposure to die with these gases. Evidently, gas concentrations should be continuously monitored and death should be confirmed in all birds prior to disposal. Dilated pupils and absence of breathing can be used as indicators of death.

CHAPTER 6

Welfare assessment methods for broiler chickens

INGRID DE JONG AND ANDY BUTTERWORTH

With increasing attention to animal welfare, the development of welfare assessment protocols for broiler chickens has become a focus of research over the past 20 years. Welfare assessment can be performed for multiple purposes: it may serve as a management tool and help farmers implement integrations to increase the welfare of their chickens; it can be used for legislation, codes of practice and quality assurance schemes; and it may help breeding companies in their choices in the selection process. Monitoring broiler welfare can provide insights into potential improvements in both welfare and production. Welfare is a part of the intrinsic quality of meat, and as such, welfare could and probably should be considered important for farmers as well as processing plants and their customers, including consumers. Welfare assessment tools may also have functions other than systematic monitoring. As an example, understanding impacts on the animals can assist the development of new housing systems and determine the effect of these systems on the welfare of the broiler chicken. As an example, for layers, the new housing system 'Rondeel' in the Netherlands has been approved and awarded three stars by the Animal Protection Organisation because of the results of welfare assessments using the Welfare Quality® layer assessment protocol (Van Niekerk, personal communication).

EFSA (2012) identified the need to monitor trends in major issues in broiler welfare in commercial flocks, to assess welfare problems and to establish whether anticipated improvements were genuine and sustainable. The EU broiler directive (Council Directive 2007/43/EC), published in 2007, highlighted that animal welfare should be monitored to guarantee at least minimal requirements. According to the directive the competent authority in each EU country was (and continues to be) directed to provide trigger (alarm) levels (animal or slaughterhouse data) based on post-mortem inspection to identify possible indications of poor welfare (Butterworth et al., 2016). Butterworth et al. (2016) carried out an inventory in EU member states and found that, at that time, only a few measures were collected post-mortem in all countries (for example, rejections, dead-on-arrival and hock burns), whereas the majority of welfare-related measures were only recorded in a few countries (for example, wing fractures, scratches, breast and joint lesions). This indicated that more harmonisation in scoring and assessment methodologies was necessary for wide and harmonised implementation. To assist the introduction of standardised animal welfare indicators, EFSA (2012) provided a list of animal-based measures indicative of broiler welfare, of which a number could be collected ante- or post-mortem in the slaughter plant, which was also confirmed by the study of Butterworth et al. (2016). Especially for broiler chickens, the combination of welfare assessment with visual meat inspection offers great potential for assessment. Broiler production cycles are relatively short which implies that remedial measures at farm level can be affected in the next production cycle; all birds pass the slaughter line, and dead birds can be assessed without negative effects on the birds (stress due to handling) and with high efficiency. In addition, assessment of birds 'on the line' offers the potential for automation of that assessment. Some of the welfare measures suggested by EFSA (2012) were already included in the Welfare Quality® broiler assessment protocol that was published in the 2009 Welfare Quality protocols (Welfare Quality, 2009). However, EFSA (2012) also indicated that for pain, frustration, boredom, and positive and negative emotional state, measures were lacking, and that further research was needed.

In this chapter we provide a summary of the current state of broiler welfare assessment methods, and examples of possible applications of these protocols, and we identify trends that will without doubt lead to improvements of protocols and a wider application in the near future. However, it is important to consider that for broiler chickens the existing protocols, despite the fact that these can be improved, can already be applied in practice. For a few indicators this is done already. For example, mortality should be monitored because of the requirements of the EU broiler directive, and several countries have already implemented standard monitoring of footpad dermatitis and hock burn at the slaughter plant (Butterworth et al., 2016).

From resource-based to animal-based measures of welfare

Initially, before the Welfare Quality® (WQ) project developed their assessment protocols for various species, the welfare of farmed animals was generally monitored by recording of resource- or management-based measures. Examples are: recording of housing dimensions, presence of resources (number of feeders, drinkers, perches, and so on), lighting schedules, light intensity, feeding schedules, temperature and ventilation programmes and biosecurity provision. These measures can be derived from management software (for example, temperature schedules) or documentation that is present on the farm, and the 'data' can be collected in a relatively short time and require relatively little training of assessors. If there is an established link between resources present in the environment or specific management practices and animal welfare, monitoring these management and resource-based measures may provide an idea of the risks for animal welfare (De Mol et al., 2006). However, resource and management-based measures cannot guarantee the welfare of the animals. Even with more or less standardised management practices there will be differences between individual farmers in the outcomes for the animals which they farm. Dependent on animal characteristics, such as genetics, early experiences and temperament, animals will perceive the environment and management in a different way. With the WQ project, this was perceived as a weakness of the previous reliance on recording resource- and management-based measures and it was decided to base the welfare assessment on animal-based measures where this was possible (Blokhuis et al., 2013).

Existing welfare assessment protocols for broiler chickens

In 2009, the European WQ project published welfare assessment protocols for various species, including for broiler chickens on-farm (Welfare Quality, 2009). This was the first set of assessment protocols that focused on animal-based measures as much as was possible, and where resource-based measures were only included when animal-based indicators were absent or too time consuming to be feasible to collect on farms. The WQ protocols were based on the 'Five Freedoms', which regard welfare as multidimensional, including freedom from suffering, a high level of biological functioning, and existence of positive experiences, and aimed to cover all different aspects of animal welfare (Blokhuis et al.,

2013). The basis for the protocols for the different species is 'domains' of welfare – four welfare principles (good feeding, good housing, good health, appropriate behaviour), and 12 welfare criteria. For each species, specific measures for each welfare criterion were developed (see Table 6.1 for the broiler measures on-farm). WQ further developed mathematical calculation methods to calculate one 'final score' for broiler welfare on-farm, with four flock welfare categories (from 'not classified' to 'excellent'). The WQ protocol is designed to be applied once per flock cycle, between 5 and 1 days before depopulation of the flock. This is because it is assumed that broiler welfare is at its worst level just before depopulation (Welfare Quality, 2009; Blokhuis et al., 2013).

A few years after the release of the WQ protocols, the European AWIN project developed an alternative to the WQ broiler assessment protocol for on-farm welfare, which aimed to be much quicker and thus more feasible to carry out in practice. The AWIN protocol also consists of animal-based measures (see Table 6.2). These are not scored on a sample of individual birds per broiler house as is done in the WQ broiler protocol but recorded when walking a predefined path in the broiler house (called a 'transect'). A smartphone and tablet application ('iWatch-Broiler') was developed to score a flock, and to enable benchmarking with other flocks that have been scored using the same method. The transect method to assess broiler welfare only scores the prevalence of the different welfare issues and the AWIN protocol does not include a calculation method to assign one welfare score to a broiler flock. The authors of the AWIN transect method indicated that the AWIN protocol can be applied as an 'early warning system' by applying it at an early age, for example, from 3 weeks of age onwards, so that a farmer would be able to take remedial measures in case any welfare issues are found (Marchewka et al., 2013; Estevez et al., 2017; BenSassi et al., 2019b).

Private initiatives have developed their own assessment protocols, and we mention one example here. RSPCA (UK and international) published their assessment protocols for various species, called 'AssureWel', including broiler chickens on-farm (RSPCA, 2018). While some of the measures that have been included are similar to WQ and the AWIN protocol, they also include additional or different measures. For example, bird distribution was included in the assessment for broiler chickens. It is important to note that the various welfare assessment protocols that are applied in practice all work towards the same goal: improving welfare of the chickens. Protocols will always differ between initiatives (on national or private level) and will be subject to change, based on the practical experience of the scheme, development of new assessment methods, and the requirements of stakeholders. The examples we will highlight in the current chapter will therefore also be subject to change in the future.

WQ also published a separate assessment protocol for broiler welfare during the end-of-life stage, including the catching of broiler chickens in the house, transport, and stunning and killing at the slaughter plant. Although the measures were defined, WQ did not publish the integration method to calculate a final flock score for the welfare level during this end-of-life stage (Welfare Quality, 2009). More recently, Jacobs et al. (2017) published the WellTrans assessment protocol that included an adjusted set of measures indicative of broiler welfare during the end-of-life stage, and which also included a method to calculate one final flock score for the welfare level during this stage.

The measures included in the WQ on-farm broiler protocol, AWIN Transect method and WellTrans assessment protocol for the end-of-life stage are discussed in more detail below, including experiences with application in practice.

Welfare Quality® broiler assessment protocol on-farm

Table 6.1 shows the various measures of the WQ on-farm broiler assessment protocol. Since its development in 2009, it has been applied in research projects in various countries such as Belgium, Brazil, the Netherlands, Spain and Norway (de Jong et al., 2016; Federici et al.,

2016; Buijs et al., 2017; Vasdal et al., 2018). Table 6.1 also provides the sample size for the different measures included in the protocol. For the scoring methodology, we refer to the assessment protocol, which is available online (www.welfarequality.net). For a couple of measures, a representative sample of broiler chickens should be selected from the broiler house and each broiler needs to be inspected individually (Table 6.1). This manual handling, or close observation of individual animals, is a feature of outcome-based assessment – and implies that it is relatively time consuming to apply the protocol in practice (de Jong et al., 2016). Assessing a sample of a minimum of 100 broiler chickens for clinical inspection (footpad dermatitis, hock burn, breast blisters, cleanliness) and another sample of 150 chickens at least for gait score means that about 2.5 hours per flock is necessary for these measures only. It is important that a representative sample of the house is taken, which means that samples should be taken from areas close to the walls and in the central area of the house between feeders and drinkers (BenSassi et al., 2019a). It is also important that the broiler chickens are selected in such a way that the sample is representative for that flock – for example, when catching the birds at random by hand, there is a risk that only the less-mobile birds are caught and that the more active and agile birds will escape from selection. It is therefore advised to use a catching pen to enclose a representative subsample of birds, and then to score each and every bird that is caught in the catching pen. Figure 6.1 shows an example of a catching pen and individual scoring of broiler chickens. In addition to the individual scoring of birds, some measures are scored at flock level, and a few are collected when the birds are sent to slaughter (see Table 6.1). Training is required to apply the WQ procedures on-farm to assure inter- and intra-observer reliability. The WQ network has developed a training and examination program for assessors (www.welfarequality.net).

Table 6.1 Measures included in the on-farm assessment protocol for broiler chickens as developed by Welfare Quality (Welfare Quality, 2009) and the respective sample size/level of assessment.

Principle	Criterion	Measure	Sample size/level
Good feeding	Absence of prolonged hunger	Proportion of emaciated broilers	Flock level (measured at the slaughterhouse)
	Absence of prolonged thirst	Drinker space	Flock level
Good housing	Comfort around resting	Plumage cleanliness	Sample of at least 100 individually inspected birds*
		Litter quality	At least 5 locations in the house
		Dust sheet test	1 location in the house
	Thermal comfort	Proportion of broilers showing panting or huddling	Flock level
	Ease of movement	Stocking density	Flock level
	Absence of injuries	Lameness	Sample of at least 150 individually scored broilers
		Footpad dermatitis	Sample of at least 100 individually inspected birds*
		Hock burn	Sample of at least 100 individually inspected birds*
		Breast blisters	Sample of at least 100 individually inspected birds*

Principle	Criterion	Measure	Sample size/level
Good health	Absence of disease	On-farm mortality	Flock level
		Culls on farm	Flock level
		Rejections for reason of disease	Flock level, registered at the slaughter plant
	Absence of pain induced by management procedures	Not applicable	
Appropriate behaviour	Expression of social behaviours	No measure developed for broiler chickens	
	Expression of other behaviours	Free range use	Flock level
		Cover on the range	Flock level
	Good human-animal relationship	Touch test	Flock level, assessed at between 12–21 locations
	Positive emotional state	Qualitative behaviour assessment	Flock level

Note: *These measures are scored in the same sample of at least 100 birds that are individually inspected.

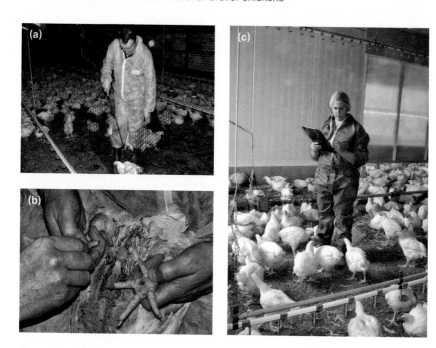

Figure 6.1 (a) Example of use of a catching pen to collect a sample of birds. Here, broilers' gait scores were determined by letting the birds walk out of the pen one-by-one. The stick is used to gently stimulate the bird to walk out of the pen. (b) Inspection of the feet to score footpad dermatitis. The same broiler is inspected for cleanliness (breast and belly area), breast blisters and hock burn. (c) Some measures are collected at flock level, such as the proportion of broilers showing panting or huddling, or the Qualitative Behaviour Assessment.

The full WQ broiler assessment protocol on-farm takes about 3–4 hours per flock. Stakeholders indicated that this could be too long for application in practice. Therefore, it has been studied whether or not the protocol could be reduced without compromising its quality. De Jong et al. (2016) assessed more than 150 broiler flocks of different strains (fast- and slower-growing) and determined relationships between the various measures. Their study indicated that there could be two ways of reducing the time to carry out the full protocol. First, footpad dermatitis, hock burn and breast irritation could be assessed in the slaughter plant (Figure 6.2) and this is currently done in many countries because of welfare regulations. When these measures are collected at the plant, the data can be used instead of assessing each individual bird on the farm, which saves time. However, cleanliness, which is measured at the same time as footpad dermatitis, hock burn and breast irritation, still needs to be assessed by inspecting at least 100 birds on-farm, thus, this will not lead to a major reduction of the time needed to carry out the protocol. Alternatively, these authors found that hock burn scores and gait score were correlated. This could mean that gait scores could be predicted from hock burn scores, which could save 1.5 hours per flock. It was proposed in this publication that further study of this relationship was needed to determine whether indeed hock burn scores can be used to predict gait score of a flock.

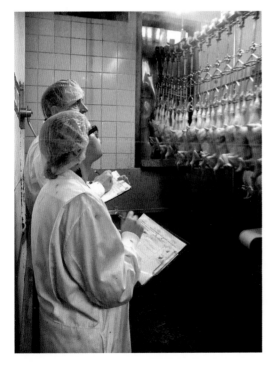

Figure 6.2 Some welfare indicators, such as hock burn, can be collected at slaughter of the birds.

Because the WQ assessment protocol has been applied in many flocks in several countries, its advantages and disadvantages have been discussed in various scientific papers. Generally speaking, most researchers feel that the majority of the measures included are valid and feasible. Some doubts have been raised with respect to the touch test, that assesses fear of humans. Results of the assessment of 50 flocks in Norway showed that the results of the touch test were related to the walking ability of the broiler flock, and it was suggested that walking ability could be a confounding factor in this score (Vasdal et al., 2018). Further, researchers doubted whether the Qualitative Behaviour Assessment (QBA) can be considered a valid measure of broiler flock behaviour. In contrast to other species, where the QBA has been validated, this has not been done for broiler chickens. Therefore, researchers have suggested that improvement of the measures in the principle 'appropriate behaviour' is necessary (de Jong et al., 2015). Finally, it has been questioned whether or not the number of birds per drinker is a valid measure for absence of prolonged thirst (de Jong et al., 2015). Although an animal-based measure of thirst has been developed (Vanderhasselt et al., 2014) researchers considered this specific test to be too time consuming to include in the protocol. Researchers have continued to work on further improvement of the protocol, for example, with respect to the behavioural measures (de Jong et al., in press) but this has thus far not led to adjusted measures.

As indicated above, WQ also provides a method to calculate a flock welfare score based on the individual measures included in the protocol. Buijs et al. (2017) determined whether the WQ flock score calculation was able to discriminate between flocks within the same housing system that differed in scores for individual welfare measures. They concluded that two measures had a very large effect on the final flock score (stocking density, and drinker space) and that the current calculation method for a final flock score showed insufficient discriminative capacity. Therefore, an adjustment of the classification system was required.

To conclude, the WQ broiler assessment protocol can be a valuable tool to assess broiler welfare on-farm. It provides detailed data on the prevalence of important welfare issues, although especially with respect to the principle 'appropriate behaviour' it is advised that further work is required to develop alternative or additional measures. With respect to the method to calculate a final flock score, the current method is considered not suitable and needs to be revised.

The transect method to assess broiler welfare on-farm

The transect method has been developed to provide an assessment protocol that is feasible to carry out in practice, because it takes limited time to assess a whole flock and can easily be learned by, for example, farmers or inspection bodies. Table 6.2 provides an overview of the measures that are included. By using a pre-defined walking path in a broiler house (a transect) the assessor scores each bird that shows one or more of the welfare issues defined in Table 6.2. Transect paths are limited by feeder and drinker lines and should include walls and the central area in the broiler house (Marchewka et al., 2013). BenSassi et al. (2019a) determined that the optimal sampling method was two transects, one near the wall and one in the central area, separated by three transects in between. The transect method takes about 45 minutes per flock and is thus more feasible to apply in practice than the WQ assessment protocol. Further, it has been shown that the transect method can be used when the broilers are as young as 3 weeks of age, and thus also be a management support tool for the farmer. An application has been developed for smartphone or tablet (iWatchBroiler) which enables benchmarking between flocks (BenSassi et al., 2019b).

Because of the method applied, that is, scoring each bird with a welfare issue each time it is observed when walking the transects, it is advised to use the transect method as a measure of 'iceberg indicators' (iceberg indicators are hypothesised outcome-based indicators of animal welfare that provide an 'overall assessment of welfare' through their ability to

Table 6.2 Measures included in the transect method to assess broiler welfare on commercial farms (Marchewka et al., 2013).

Measure	Definition
Immobile	No attempt to move, even after slight encouragement
Limping	Visual signs of severe uneven walk
Dirty	Side and back feathers visibly dirty
Sick	Clear signs of impaired health, such as feather ruffling, watery eyes, pale comb, usually resting
Agonizing	The bird lays on the floor with closed eyes, breathing with difficulty
Dead	

effectively summarise many different alternative measures of welfare). An iceberg measure does not provide the exact level (percentage of incidence) of welfare issues in a broiler flock, but by observing a number of flocks and benchmarking it can be used to identify flocks that are at risk for developing welfare problems. If needed, more detailed observations may follow the inspection using the transect method to identify causes of the problem and apply remedial measures. Further, it should be noted that the transect method in its current stage does not include behavioural indicators of broiler welfare, and thus only includes a limited set of welfare indicators.

WellTrans assessment of broiler chicken welfare during the end-of-life stage

In addition to the on-farm stage, the procedures around thinning/depopulation and slaughter of broiler chickens have associated welfare risks. Broilers are caught, either by catching machines or by hand, loaded into crates or containers, transported, kept waiting in a lairage at the slaughter plant, and subsequently unloaded, stunned and killed. Although within WQ measures were defined to assess welfare during the end-of life stage (Welfare Quality, 2009), this slaughter protocol has never been tested on a large scale, and no mathematical calculation for a 'one flock welfare score' has been developed for the slaughter section. Recently, the WellTrans method to assess welfare during the end-of-life phase has been developed and tested in Belgian broiler flocks (Jacobs et al., 2017). Table 6.3 shows the measures that are included in the WellTrans welfare assessment protocol; these are all assessed on arrival

Table 6.3 Measures included in the WellTrans protocol to assess broiler welfare at slaughter (Jacobs et al., 2017). For detailed instructions to assess the birds, see Jacobs et al. (2017).

Measure	Sample size
Panting or huddling in the lorry	60 transport containers inspected on the lorry/in lairage (front, middle, back of the lorry)
Trapped limbs, heads, toes	60 transport containers, at the same time as panting/huddling
Splayed legs	60 containers as defined above
Broilers (partially) sitting or standing on each other	60 containers as defined above
Supine birds	60 containers as defined above
Wing fractures	Prevalence during an observation period of 10 minutes at the slaughter line, after plucking
Leg fractures	Identical to wing fractures, same sample
Bruises	Prevalence by observing the number of whole carcasses showing bruises at the slaughter line, after plucking
Dead-on-arrival	As recorded by the slaughter plant
Rejection percentage	Rejections because of disease or quality, as recorded by the slaughter plant

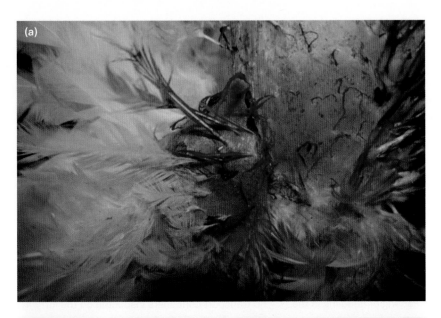

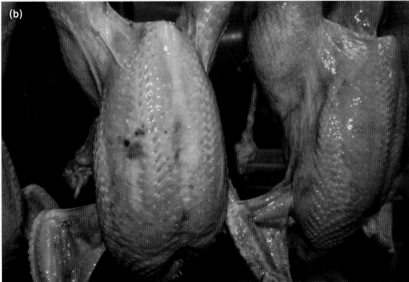

Figure 6.3 Examples of welfare issues that may occur as a consequence of pre-slaughter procedures in broiler chickens: (a) wing fracture; (b) bruise.

of the broilers at the slaughter plant (see Figure 6.3 for examples). Total time to assess all indicators (Table 6.3) has been estimated to be less than 1 hour per flock. Broiler welfare experts were invited to provide scores for the different welfare aspects, and based on these a single flock score was developed. The WellTrans protocol does not include measures related to stunning and killing procedures. WQ does include some of these indicators but as indicated earlier, the WQ assessment protocol for the end-of-life phase needs further improvement, and this remains to be done in the future.

Benchmarking and feedback to farmers

Standardised welfare assessment protocols offer the potential for benchmarking of farms or flocks. This can not only provide insight into the actual welfare level of a flock in comparison to other flocks for the integrator, slaughter plant or customer, but can also provide the farmer with insight into the actual performance of his/her flock in relation to other flocks in similar production systems. To enable benchmarking, quick feedback to farmers and a clear and easy-to-read overview of their performance is essential. The AWIN project developed their smartphone application in such a way that it enables benchmarking with other, previous flocks on the same farm, but such applications can easily be used to benchmark flocks with respect to other flocks of, for example, the same company or integrator. In a study in the Netherlands in 2013–2014, a sample of broiler farms was visited four times over a period of 4 years. Farmers were provided with a report on their results and the average results for all farms visited (within the same production system) to enable benchmarking. Farmers indicated that this benchmarking was one of the advantages of systematic welfare monitoring, and that it is essential to provide a quick and clear feed-back on their performance to stimulate them to improve the next flocks (if necessary). They, however, also indicated that it is also essential to assist them with management advice in order to improve their performance (de Jong et al., 2015).

Automation

The welfare assessment protocols described above are all based on manual and visual assessment of the various welfare indicators. However, with the current development of automated methods to assess welfare, automation offers the potential for feasible and (more) objective assessment of broiler flock welfare. When applied continuously, automated measures can also provide an early warning of disease and welfare issues, and be used as a management tool by farmers (BenSassi et al., 2016). Here we give some examples of automated tools for welfare assessment, but it is clear that with the current rate of developments in technologies there will be many more opportunities in the future that will provide opportunity for large-scale monitoring. Further, the trends towards automation of welfare assessment also raise the question how to handle the large amount of data that will be provided by these systems, for example, in relation to privacy legislation and ownership but also in relation to interpretation. Thus, there is not only a need to develop automated tools for welfare assessment, but also develop algorithms to assist farmers and others in the interpretation of the data that are collected.

Camera vision techniques are currently applied to record measures like footpad dermatitis, hock burn and bruises at the slaughter plant (for example, de Jong et al., 2008) (Figure 6.4). Such systems have already been used at slaughter plants for several years, and recent developments in techniques will without doubt lead to more indicators being recorded at the plant. The vision system is linked to software that calculates welfare scores used, for example for regulatory purposes. Camera vision techniques have also been developed to record welfare issues on-farm. For example, Aydin (2017) used camera vision techniques and developed algorithms to score lameness in broiler chickens in the house. The advantage when compared to human assessment is that these systems can score lameness continuously and thus might also be used to generate early warning signals for the farmer. Camera vision systems and the optical flow technique have shown to be able to record footpad dermatitis in the broiler house (Dawkins et al., 2017). However, until

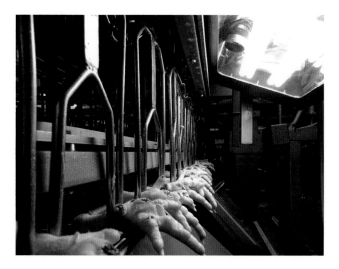

Figure 6.4 Camera vision system to score footpad lesions at the slaughter plant (photo: Meyn Food Processing Technology B.V.).

now, these systems are not in widespread use in practice, probably due to the relatively high costs that are involved with installing them. In addition to vision systems, recent research also focuses on sensor techniques to measure activity and location of the broilers in the house (van der Sluis et al., 2019). Nowadays these techniques are in the validation phase and further development will be necessary before these can be applied on commercial farms.

Conclusion

Broiler welfare assessment will help to improve on-farm welfare. Various assessment protocols have been developed, and recent developments in technology will without doubt lead to increased application of welfare assessment protocols in practice. In this chapter we describe examples of assessment protocols that can be applied in practice, although further improvement of these protocols is still necessary.

CHAPTER 7

What can we do to improve broiler welfare?

CHARLOTTE BERG, JOY MENCH, ANDY BUTTERWORTH
AND INGRID DE JONG

If broiler welfare is to be improved, a number of different approaches have to be combined. The term 'improvement' indicates that something is suboptimal or even poor; a level from which it can then be improved. However, improvements can still be made from a starting position which is acceptable, or at least in compliance with the relevant broiler or broiler breeder welfare legislation. It could also be possible to 'improve' broiler welfare to a level where the general quality of life of the birds is really good, where positive experiences become an essential aspect.

In any case, to achieve improvements, we need to identify suitable areas for improvement (Figure 7.1). To do this, we must have knowledge about the biological needs of the birds, at different stages of life. In this book the previous chapters have, in line with this, dealt with animal

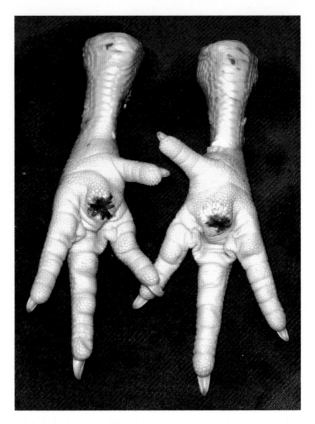

Figure 7.1 To be able to evaluate broiler welfare improvements, systematic assessments have to be carried out before and after any kind of intervention which aims to improve the welfare of the birds. The photo shows broiler feet ready for inspection and classification with respect to footpad dermatitis.

welfare as a concept, the link between health and welfare, how housing and management relates to broiler welfare, various welfare assessment methods and so on. The reason for this focus on a range of topics, is, of course, that in order to achieve improvement, we must first identify problem areas or suboptimal areas in relation to the birds' welfare status, understand why these problems have arisen, identify causal factors and map often complex correlations, suggest possible solutions and later follow these up as part of a systematic evaluation. Quantification is an inherent aspect of improvement; without at least an attempt at quantifying the extent of a given broiler welfare problem it will be impossible to know if interventions and actions taken will have had the desired (hopefully positive) effect, that is, if increased bird welfare has actually been achieved. Such quantification means that indicators or measures, and usually a combination of different (that is, more than 1) indicators, have to be chosen, shown to be valid as measures of welfare, and standardised, to allow realistic assessment of the welfare state of the birds. Such assessment schemes do exist (see Chapter 6), but different schemes may emphasise different aspects of broiler welfare and the choice of indicators must be based on the issues in question.

In summary, there are three major areas influencing broiler welfare, which all need attention to optimise the welfare of the birds. These are breeding and genetics, housing and feeding, and management and care.

It is generally acknowledged that the genetics of the modern broiler does contribute to some of the welfare problems that can be seen today. Breeding and genetic selection have changed the conformation of the broiler, which is now a heavy bird with a high growth rate and proportionally larger breast muscle mass. This, in turn, has increased the risk for impaired walking ability and metabolic problems such as ascites and SDS. The breeding companies are of course aware of this, and health and welfare aspects are certainly included in their breeding programmes. These goals must nevertheless be balanced against production goals, for monetary reasons. Having said this, neither the producers nor the breeding companies benefit from birds becoming sick or having to be culled/dying prematurely, instead of entering the food chain. In parallel with the creation of very fast-growing strains, there has also been genetic selection for lines of birds which focus on breeding for birds less prone to various welfare problems, and a trend towards development of slow-growing broiler strains for a niche market (Figure 7.2). These birds are generally less prone to leg pathologies, lameness and other problems related to rapid growth. However, because of the longer rearing period

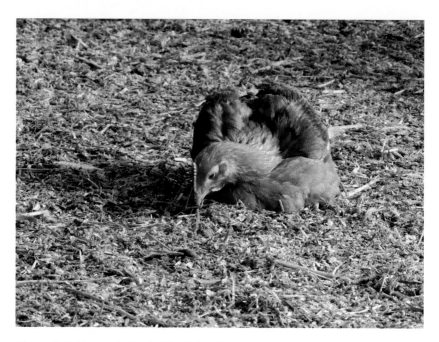

Figure 7.2 Slow-growing broiler hybrids have been developed to decrease the risk of, for example, gait abnormalities.

and lower food conversion rate they are also usually more expensive to produce and hence less affordable for certain consumer groups.

Traditionally, much focus in relation to broiler welfare has been placed on housing, as this is an area that has caused much concern over the years. Some examples of the link between house conditions and welfare are: (1) overstocking, which can result in restricted movement, and constantly interrupted rest; and (2) poor ventilation, resulting in over-heating and poor air quality including high ammonia and dust levels, as well as poor litter quality which can then result in contact dermatitis and soiled plumage. Many areas of broiler farm housing design have been the subject of research projects, enforcement interest by legislators and campaign attention from animal welfare NGOs. Legislation and private and industry standards have been designed to prevent the most extreme housing designs and farming systems, with limits to stocking densities, improved ceiling height and improved ventilation capacity, better water systems which reduce spillage, improvements in water quality, and a requirement that there are at least a minimum (6 hours in many countries) number of hours of darkness per 24 hour cycle. This has led to improvements in many countries and at many farms, but much work still remains, and broiler production is in many cases still a very intensive, and potentially welfare challenging, form of animal husbandry.

Broiler feed composition and quality have a considerable impact on broiler growth rate, skeleton formation, gut health and faecal consistency, thereby affecting broiler welfare in several ways. The temporal and spatial distribution of feed has an impact on the birds' welfare. For example, meal feeding or *ad libitum* (free) access feeding, feeder distribution in the shed, and the use of scatter feeding to activate the birds will all influence the birds' behaviour and welfare.

There are different types of 'alternative' broiler production methods practised in various regions, and to suit the demands of various consumer groups; these include organic standards (Figure 7.3), outdoor free-range production (Figure 7.4), use of alternative feed ingredients etcetera. Although novel hybrids are often used in these systems, the conventional high growth potential broiler genotypes (Aviagen, Cobb) nevertheless completely dominate the global market.

The structure of the broiler industry varies between countries and regions with respect to farm size, ownership structure and the level of integration. One can sometimes get the impression that genetics, housing, feed composition, and so on, are all completely steered and directed by the breeding companies, the feed mills, the company/integrators and the slaughterhouses, and that the individual producer or the staff can do very little to influence the welfare of the birds. This is simply not correct.

A skilled and knowledgeable stockperson can help by mitigating the negative influence of several of the factors mentioned above, and can

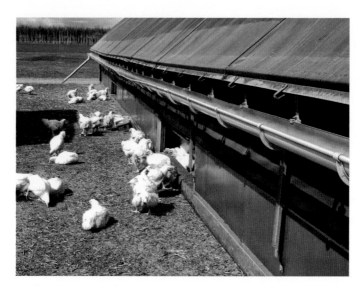

Figure 7.3 Organic broiler production in mobile sheds.

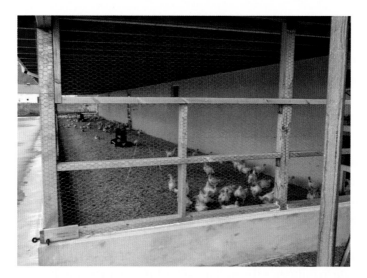

Figure 7.4 Broiler production in a system where the birds are allowed to go outside, but still kept within rather strict biosecurity barriers, that is, without contact with soil or wildlife.

also actively put pressure on the various suppliers of day-old chicks, feed, equipment and also on catching staff, thereby decreasing the welfare risks and improving bird welfare. A skilled stockperson takes responsibility for maintaining strict biosecurity standards and adhering to vaccination recommendations. A skilled stockperson can at an early stage detect problems related to bird health and rapidly take whatever action is needed, including seeking veterinary advice or humanely culling sick or injured birds. A skilled stockperson (Figure 7.5) will notice also minor changes in bird behaviour and adjust ventilation, accordingly, will notice small changes in water and feed consumption and take appropriate action, and will be able to prevent major bird welfare problems from occurring.

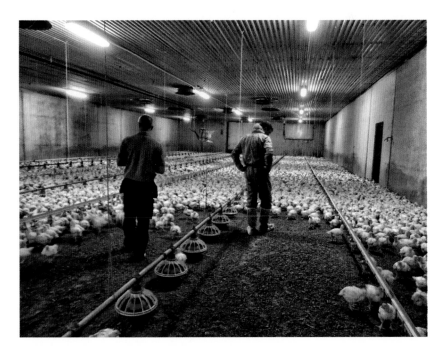

Figure 7.5 A skilled and knowledgeable stockperson, with the support of professional advisers from the veterinary and the production sector, is a crucial prerequisite for good broiler welfare on the farm.

How can good stockpersonship be achieved? Running a broiler farm requires a wide range of skills and competencies, including logistics, mechanics and equipment maintenance, transport, computer software management, animal science, economy, poultry nutrition, staff management and often also crop production and some commercial marketing. Nobody can be expected to master these fields without proper education and training. Hence, relevant basic education and also continuous professional development courses focused on poultry production should be available in order to ensure that current and future generations can rear broilers in a way that satisfies consumer demands, food safety expectations and animal welfare requirements. Proper training and good knowledge of the birds' physiological, nutritional and behavioural needs is a prerequisite, but in practice, there also has to be a genuine personal interest in the birds, and in good standards of house environment and animal care. It is that 'eye for birds' that is so difficult to pinpoint in research but that nevertheless makes a 'good stockperson' good, and potentially makes a huge difference from a bird welfare perspective.

References

Abeyesinghe, S.M., Wathes, C.M., Nicol, C.J. and Randall, J.M. (2001) The aversion of broiler chickens to concurrent vibrational and thermal stressors. *Applied Animal Behaviour Science* 73, 199–215.

Al-Homidan, A., Robertson, J.F. and Petchey, A.M. (2003). Review of the effect of ammonia and dust concentrations on broiler performance. *World's Poultry Science Journal* 59, 340–349.

Alleman, F. and Leclercq, B (1997) Effect of dietary protein and environmental temperature on growth performance and water consumption of male broiler chickens. *British Poultry Science* 38(5), 607–610.

Alvino, G.M., Blatchford, R.A., Archer G.S. and Mench, J.A. (2009) Light intensity during rearing affects the behavioural synchrony and resting patterns of broiler chickens. *British Poultry Science* 50(3), 275–283.

Anderson, D.P., Beard, C.W. and Hanson, R.P. (1966) Influence of poultry house dust, ammonia and carbon dioxide on the resistance of chickens to Newcastle disease virus. *Avian Diseases* 10, 177–188.

Archer, G. (2017) Exposing broiler eggs to green, red and white light during incubation. *Animal* 11(7), 1203–1209.

Aviagen (2018) Ross parent stock handbook. Available at: http://en.aviagen.com/assets/Tech_Center/Ross_PS/RossPSHandBook2018.pdf (accessed 7 May 2019).

Aydin, A. (2017) Development of an early detection system for lameness of broilers using computer vision. *Computers and Electronics in Agriculture* 136, 140–146.

Aziz, T. (2010) Harmful effects of ammonia on birds. *Poultry World*. Available at: https://www.poultryworld.net/Breeders/Health/2010/10/Harmful-effects-of-ammonia-on-birds-WP008071W/ (accessed 8 August 2019).

BenSassi, N., Averos, X. and Estevez, I. (2016) Technology and poultry welfare. *Animals: an open access journal from MDPI* 6.

BenSassi, N., Averos, X. and Estevez, I. (2019a) Broiler chickens on-farm welfare assessment: estimating the robustness of the transect sampling method. *Frontiers in Veterinary Science* 6(98), 522–532.

BenSassi, N., Averos, X. and Estevez, I. (2019b) The potential of the transect method for early detection of welfare problems in broiler chickens. *Poultry Science* 98, 522–532.

Berg, C. (2004) Pododermatitis and hock burn in broiler chickens. In: Weeks, C.A. and Butterworth, A. (eds) *Measuring and Auditing Broiler Welfare*. CABI Publishing, Wallingford, pp. 37–49.

Berg, C. (2012) The need for monitoring farm animal welfare during mass killing for disease eradication purposes. *Animal Welfare* 21, 357–361.

Blokhuis, H., Miele, M., Veissier, I. and Jones, B. (eds) (2013) *Improving Farm Animal Welfare: Science and Society Working Together: the Welfare Quality Approach*. Wageningen Academic Publishers, Wageningen.

Bokkers, E.A.M. and Koene, P. (2003) Behaviour of fast- and slow growing broilers to 12 weeks of age and the physical consequences. *Applied Animal Behaviour Science* 81, 59–72.

Buijs, S., Ampe, B. and Tuyttens, F.A.M. (2017) Sensitivity of the Welfare Quality® broiler chicken protocol to differences between intensively reared indoor flocks: which factors explain overall classification? *Animal* 11, 244–253.

Butterworth, A., de Jong, I.C., Keppler, C., Knierim, U., Stadig, L. and Lambton, S. (2016) What is being measured, and by whom? Facilitation of communication on technical measures among competent authorities in the implementation of the European Union Broiler Directive (2007/43/EC). *Animal* 10, 302–308.

Butterworth, A., Reeves, N.A., Harbour, D., Werret, G. and Kestin, S.C. (2001) Molecular typing of strains of Staphylococcus aureus isolated from bone and joint lesions in lame broilers by random amplification of polymorphic DNA. *Poultry Science* 45: 35–42.

Butterworth, A. and Weeks, C. (2010) The impact of disease on welfare. In: Duncan, I.J.H. and Hawkins, P. (eds) *The Welfare of Domestic Fowl and Other Captive Birds*. Springer, Dordrecht, pp. 189–218.

Casadio, M., Massi, P., Tosi, G., Fiorentini, L., Taddei, R., Bolognesi, P. and Catelli, M. (2014) Evaluation of the level of bacterial contamination of eggs and dead-in-shell chicks in an industrial chicken hatchery. *Large Animal Review* 20(3), 119–123.

Castellini, C., Mugnai, C., Moscati, L., Mattioli, S., Amato, M.G., Mancinelli, A.C. and Dal Bosco, A. (2016) Adaptation to organic rearing system of eight different chicken genotypes: behaviour, welfare and performance. *Italian Journal of Animal Science* 15, 37–46.

Council Directive 2007/43/EC of 28 June 2007 laying down minimum rules for the protection of chickens kept for meat production. *Official Journal of the European Union* L182, 19–28.

Council Regulation (EC) No 1099/2009 of 24 September 2009 on the protection of animals at the time of killing. *Official Journal of the European Union* L303, 1–30.

David, B., Moe, R.O., Michel, V., Lund, V. and Mejdell, C. (2015a) Air quality in alternative housing systems may have an impact on laying hen welfare. Part I – dust. *Animals* 5, 495–511.

David, B., Mejdell, C., Michel, V., Lund, V. and Moe, R.O. (2015b) Air quality in alternative housing systems may have an impact on laying hen welfare. Part II – ammonia. *Animals* 5, 886–896.

Dawkins, M.S. (2018) Stocking density: can we judge how much space poultry need? In: Mench, J.A. (ed.) *Advances in Poultry Welfare*. Woodhead Publishing, Cambridge, pp. 227–242.

Dawkins, M.S., Cook, P.A., Whittingham, M.J., Mansell, K.A. and Harper, A.E. (2003) What makes free-range broiler chickens range? In situ measurement of habitat preference. *Animal Behaviour* 66, 151–160.

Dawkins, M.S., Roberts, S.J., Cain, R.J., Nickson, T. and Donnelly, C.A. (2017) Early warning of footpad dermatitis and hockburn in broiler chicken flocks using optical flow, bodyweight and water consumption. *Veterinary Record* 180, 499.

D'Eath, R.B., Tolkamp, B.J., Kyriazakis, I. and Lawrence, A.B. (2009) 'Freedom from hunger' and preventing obesity: the animal welfare implications of reducing food quantity or quality. *Animal Behaviour* 77, 275–288.

Deep, A., Raginski, C., Schwean-Lardner, K., Fancher, B. and Classen, H.L. (2013) Minimum light intensity threshold to prevent negative effects on broiler production and welfare. *British Poultry Science* 54, 686–694.

De Jong, I.C. and van Emous, R.A. (2017) Broiler breeding flocks: management and animal welfare. In: Applegate, T. (ed.) *Sustainable Broiler Production*. Burleigh Dodds Science Publishers, Sawston, pp. 1–19

De Jong, I.C. and Guemene, D. (2011) Major welfare issues in broiler breeders. *Worlds Poulty Science Journal* 67, 73–81.

De Jong, I. C. and Swalander, M. (2012) Housing and management of broiler breeders and turkey breeders. In: Sandilands, V. and Hocking, P.M. (eds)

Alternative Systems for Poultry. Health, Welfare and Productivity. Poultry Science, Symposium Series No.(30). CABI, Oxford, pp. 225–249.

De Jong, I. C., Gerritzen, M. A., Reimert, H. G. M., Fritsma, E. and Pieterse, C. (2008) Automated measurement of foot pad lesions in broiler chickens. Proceedings of the 4th International Workshop on the Assessment of Animal Welfare at Farm and Group Level, 10–13 September 2008, Ghent, Belgium.

De Jong, I.C., Wolthuis-Fillerup, M. and van Emous, R.A. (2009) Development of sexual behaviour in commercially housed broiler breeders after mixing. *British Poultry Science* 50, 151–160.

De Jong, I.C., Perez Moya, T., Gunnink, H., Van den Heuvel, H., Hindle, V., Mul, M., Van Reenen, C.G. (2011a) Symplifying the Welfare Quality assessment protocol for broilers. Report 533, Wageningen UR Livestock Research, Lelystad.

De Jong, I.C., Van Harn, J., Gunnink, H., Hindle, V. and Lourens, S. (2011b) Incidence and severity of foot pad lesions in regular Dutch broiler flocks, Wageningen UR Livestock Research.

De Jong, I.C., van Harn, J., Gunnink, H., Hindle, V.A., Lourens, A., 2012. Footpad dermatitis in Dutch broiler flocks: prevalence and factors of influence. *Poultry Science* 91(7), 1569–1574.

De Jong, I.C., Hindle, V.A., Butterworth, A., Engel, B., Ferrari, P., Gunnink, H., Moya, T.P., Tuyttens, F.A.M. and van Reenen, C.G. (2016) Simplifying the Welfare Quality® assessment protocol for broiler chicken welfare. *Animal* 10, 117–127.

De Jong, I.C., Van Riel, J.W., Bracke, M.B.M. and van den Brand, H. (2017) A 'meta-analysis' of effects of post-hatch food and water deprivation on development, performance and welfare of chickens. *PLoS One* 12, e0189350.

De Jong, I.C., Gunnink, H., Van Hattum, T., Van Riel, J.W., Raaijmakers, M.M.P., Zoet, EL. And van den Brand (2018) Comparison of performance, health and welfare aspects between commercially housed hatchery-hatched and on-farm hatched broiler flocks, *Animal* 13, 1269–1279.

De Jong, I.C., Van Riel, J., Hoevenaar, T. and Van Niekerk, T. (2019) Possible improvement of measures within the principle 'appropriate behaviour' of the Welfare Quality® boiler assessment protocol. Wageningen Livestock Research Report 1192, https://doi.org/10.18174/499603.

De Mol, R.M., Schouten, W.G.P., Evers, E., Drost, H., Houwers, H.W.J. and Smits, A.C. (2006) A computer model for welfare assessment of poultry production systems for laying hens. *Njas-Wageningen Journal of Life Sciences* 54, 157–168.

Decuypere, E., Hocking, P.M., Tona, K., Onagbesan, O., Bruggeman, V., Jones, E.K.M., Cassy, S., Rideau, N., Metayer, S., Jego, Y., Putterflam, J., Tesseraud, S., Collin, A., Duclos, M., Trevidy, J.J. and Williams, J. (2006) Broiler breeder paradox: a project report. *Worlds Poultry Science Journal* 62, 443–453.

Donofre, A.C., Silva, I.J.O., Nazazerno, A.C. and Ferreira, I.E.D.P. (2017) Mechanical vibrations in the transport of hatching eggs and the losses caused in the hatch and quality of broiler chicks. *Journal of Agricultural Engineering* 48, 36–41.

EFSA (2010) Scientific opinion on welfare aspects of the management and housing of the grand-parent and parent stocks raised and kept for breeding purposes. *EFSA Journal* 8, 811667, https://doi.org/10.2903/j.efsa.2010.1667.

EFSA (2012) Scientific Opinion on the use of animal-based measures to assess welfare of broilers. *EFSA Journal* 10, 2774, 1–74.

Ekstrand, C., Carpenter, T.E., Andersson, I. and Algers, B. (1998) Prevalence and control of foot-pad dermatitis in broilers in Sweden. *British Poultry Science* 39, 318–324.

Estevez, I., Battini, M., Canali, E., Ruiz, R., Stilwell, G., Ferrante, V., Minero, M., Marchewka, J., Barbieri, S., Mattiello, S., de Heredia, I.B., Dwyer, C.M. and Zanella, A. (2017) AWIN mobile apps; animal welfare assessment at your fingertips. *Journal of Animal Science* 95, 6–7.

European Commission (2018) Report from the Commission to the European Parliament and the Council on the application of Directive 2007/43/EC and its influence on the welfare of chickens kept for meat production, as well as the development of welfare indicators. Available at: https://ec.europa.eu/transparency/regdoc/rep/1/2018/EN/COM-2018-181-F1-EN-MAIN-PART-1.PDF (accessed 8 August 2019).

Fanatico, A.C., Pillai, P.B., Hester, P.Y., Falcone, C., Mench, J.A., Owens, C.M. and Emmert, J.L. (2008) Performance, livability, and carcass yield of slow- and fast-growing chicken genotypes fed low-nutrient or standard diets and raised indoors or with outdoor access. *Poultry Science* 87, 1012–1021.

Fanatico, A.C., Mench, J.A., Archer, G.S., Liang, Y., Brewer Gusalsis, V.B., Owens, C.M. and Donoguhue, A.M. (2016) Effect of outdoor structural enrichments on the performance, use of range area, and behavior of organic meat chickens. *Poultry Science* 95, 1980–1988.

Federici, J.F., Vanderhasselt, R., Sans, E.C.O., Tuyttens, F.A.M., Souza, A.P.O. and Molento, C.F.M. (2016) Assessment of broiler chicken welfare in southern Brazil. *Brazilian Journal of Poultry Science* 18, 133–140.

Gebhardt-Henrich, S.G., Toscano, M.J. and Wurbel, H. (2017) Perch use by broiler breeders and its implication on health and production. *Poultry Science* 96, 3539–3549.

Gebhardt-Henrich, S.G., Toscano, M.J. and Wurbel, H. (2018) Use of aerial perches and perches on aviary tiers by broiler breeders. *Applied Animal Behaviour Science* 203, 24–33.

Gerritzen, M. and Gibson, T. (2016) Animal welfare at depopulation strategies during disease control actions. In: Velarde, A. and Raj, M. (eds) *Animal Welfare at Slaughter.* 5M Publishing, Sheffield, pp. 199–218.

Giersberg, M.F., Hartung, J., Kemper, N. and Spindler, B. (2016) Floor space covered by broiler chickens kept at stocking densities according to Council Directive 2007/43/EC. *Veterinary Record* 179, 124.

Hess, J.B., Macklin, K.S., Norton, R.A., Bilgili, S.F. and Blake, J.P. (2009) Effective broiler litter management. WATTAgNet.com. Available at: https://www.wattagnet.com/articles/764-effective-broiler-litter-management (accessed 8 August 2019).

Hiemstra, S. and Ten Napel, J. (2011) Study of the impact of genetic selection on the welfare of chickens bred and kept for meat production. Letter of Contract N° SANCO/2011/12254. Final Report. Available at: https://ec.europa.eu/food/sites/food/files/animals/docs/aw_practice_farm_broilers_653020_final-report_en.pdf (accessed 8 October 2020).

Hocking, P.M., Zaczek, V., Jones, E.K.M. and McLeod, M.G. (2004) Different concentrations and sources of dietary fibre may improve the welfare of female broiler breeders. *British Poultry Science* 45, 9-19.

Jacobs, L., Delezie , E., Goethals, K., Ampe, B., Duchateau, L. and Tuyttens, F.A.M. (2017) *Vleeskippenwelzijn tijdens de pre-slachtfase Evaluatieprotocol en Online integratie-tool.* ILVO, Melle.

James, C., Asher, L., Herborn, K. and Wiseman, J. (2018) The effect of supplementary ultraviolet wavelengths on broiler chicken welfare indicators. *Applied Animal Behaviour Science* 209, 55–64.

Jones, E.K.M., Prescott, N.B., Cook, P., White, R.P. and Wathes, C.M., (2001) Ultraviolet light and mating behaviour in domestic broiler breeders. *British Poultry Science Journal* 42, 23–32.

Jones, E.K.M., Wathes, C.A. and Webster, A.J.F. (2005) Avoidance of atmospheric ammonia by domestic fowl and the effect of early experience. *Applied Animal Behaviour Science* 90, 293–308.

Kestin, S.C., Knowles, T.G., Tinch, A.E. and Gregory, N.G. (1992) Prevalence of leg weakness in broiler chickens and its relationship with genotype. *Veterinary Record* 131, 190–194.

Kittelsen, K.E., Granquist, E.G., Kolbjornsen, O., Nafstad, O. and Moe, R.O. (2015) A comparison of post-mortem findings in broilers dead-on-farm and broilers dead-on-arrival at the abattoir. *Poultry Science* 94, 2622–2629.

Knowles, T.G., Brown, S.N., Warriss, P.D., Butterworth, A. and Hewitt, L. (2004) Welfare aspects of chick handling in broiler and laying hen hatcheries. *Animal Welfare* 13, 409–418.

Lee, K.W., Lillehoj, H.S., Lee, S.H., Jang, S.I., Ritter, G.D., Bautista, D.A. and Lillehoj, E.P. (2011) Impact of fresh or used litter on the posthatch immune system of commercial broilers. *Avian Diseases* 55, 539–544.

Leone, E.H. and Estevez, I. (2008) Economic and welfare benefits of environmental enrichment for broiler breeders. *Poultry Science* 87, 14–21.

Lerner, H. (2017) Conceptions of health and disease in plants and animals. In: Schramme, T. and Edwards, S. (eds) *Handbook of the Philosophy of Medicine*. Springer, Dordrecht, pp. 287–301.

Lewis, P.D. and Morris, T.R. (2000) Poultry and coloured light. *World's Poultry Science Journal* 56, 189–207.

Li, C., Schallier, S., Lesuisse, J., Lamberigts, C., Driessen, B., Everaert, N. and Buyse, J. (2018) The learning ability and memory retention of broiler breeders: 2 transgenerational effects of reduced balanced protein diet on reward-based learning. *Animal* 13(6), 1260–1268.

Marchewka, J., Watanabe, T.T.N., Ferrante, V. and Estevez, I. (2013) Welfare assessment in broiler farms: Transect walks versus individual scoring. *Poultry Science* 92, 2588–2599.

Millman, S.T., Duncan, I.J.H. and Widowski, T.M. (2000) Male broiler breeder fowl display high levels of aggression toward females. *Poultry Science* 79, 1233–1241.

Nääs, I.A., Graciano, D.E., Garcia, R.G., Santana, M.R. and Neves, D.P. (2014) Heat loss in one day old pullets inside a hatchery. *Engenharia Agrícola* 34(4), 610–616.

NCC (2017) National Chicken Council Animal Welfare Guidelines and Audit Checklist. Available at: https://www.nationalchickencouncil.org/wp-content/uploads/2018/07/NCC-Animal-Welfare-Guidelines_Broilers_July2018.pdf (accessed 8 August 2019).

NCC (2018) Statistics. Available at: https://www.nationalchickencouncil.org/about-the-industry/statistics/broiler-chicken-industry-key-facts/ (accessed 8 August 2019).

Nielsen, B.L., Thomsen, M.G., Sørensen, P. and Young, J.F. (2003) Feed and strain effects on the use of outdoor areas by broilers. *British Poultry Science* 44, 161–169.

Nielsen, B.L., Thodberg, K., Malmkvist, J. and Steenfeldt, S. (2011) Proportion of insoluble fibre in the diet affects behaviour and hunger in broiler breeders growing at similar rates. *Animal* 5, 1247–1258.

Olkowski, A.A., Abbott, J.A. and Classen, H.L. (2005) Pathogenesis of ascites in broilers raised at low altitude: aetiological considerations based on echocardiographic findings. *Journal of Veterinary Medicine Series A* 52(4): 166–171.

Osman, K.M., Kappell, A.D., Elhadidy, M., ElMougy, F., El-Ghany, W.A., Orabi, A., Mubarak, A.S., Dawoud, T.M., Hemeg, H.A., Moussa, I.M.I., Hessain, A.M. and Yousef, H.M.Y. (2018) Poultry hatcheries as potential reservoirs for antimicrobial-resistant Escherichia coli: a risk to public health and food safety. *Scientific Reports* 8, 5859.

Oyetunde, O.O., Thomson, R.G. and Carlson, H.C. (1978) Aerosol exposure of ammonia, dust and Eschericia coli in broiler chickens. *Canadian Veterinary Journal* 19, 187–193.

Pastor, A. (2016) Litter management – Part 1: Good litter for healthy birds. *Poultry World*. Available at: https://www.poultryworld.net/Broilers/Housing/2011/10/Litter-management--Part-1-Good-litter-for-healthy-birds-WP009463W/ (accessed 8 August 2019).

Petracci, M., Soglia, F., Madruga, M., Carvalho, L., Ida, E. and Estevez, M. (2019) Wooden-breast, white striping, and spaghetti meat: causes, consequences and consumer perception of emerging broiler meat abnormalities. *Comprehensive Reviews in Food Science and Food Safety*, doi: 10.1111/1541-4337.12431.

Raj, M. and Velarde, A. (2016) Electrical stunning and killing methods. In: Velarde, A. and Raj, M. (eds) *Animal Welfare at Slaughter.* 5m Publishing, Sheffield, pp. 111–132.

Raj, A.B.M. and O'Callaghan, M. (2001) Evaluation of a pneumatically operated captive bolt for stunning/killing broiler chickens. *British Poultry Science* 42, 295–299.

Raj, A.B.M. and O'Callaghan, M. (2004) Effect of amount and frequency of head-only stunning currents on the electroencephalograms and somatosensory evoked potentials in broilers. *Animal Welfare* 13, 159–170.

Raj, A.B.M., Wilkins, L.J., O'Callaghan, M. and Phillips, A.J. (2001) Effect of electrical stun/kill method, interval between killing and neck cutting and blood vessels cut on blood loss and meat quality in broilers. *British Poultry Science* 42, 51–56.

Reijrink, I.A.M., Meijerhof R., Kemp B. and Van Brand H. (2008) The chicken embryo and its micro environment during egg storage and early incubation. *World Poultry Science Journal* 64, 581–598.

Riber, A.B., de Jong, I.C., H.A., van de Weerd. H.A. and Steenfeldt, S. (2017) Environmental enrichment for broiler breeders: an undeveloped field. *Frontiers in Veterinary Science* 4, doi: 10.3389/fvets.2017.00086.

Riber, A.B., van de Weerd, H.A., de Jong, I.C. and Steenfeldt, S. (2018) Review of environmental enrichment for broiler chickens. *Poultry Science* 97, 378–389.

Ritz, C.W., Fairchild, B.D. and Lacy, M.P. (2017) Litter quality and broiler performance. UGA Extension Bulletin 1267. Available at: https://extension.uga.edu/publications/detail.html?number = B1267andtitle = Litter%20Quality%20and%20Broiler%20Performance (accessed 8 August 2019).

RSPCA (2017) *Welfare Standards for Hatcheries (Chicks, Poults and Ducklings)*. RSPCA, Horsham.

RSPCA (2018) *The AssureWel Manual: The AssureWel Approach to Improving Farm Animal Welfare: The Development and Use of Welfare Outcome Assessments in Farm Assurance*. RSPCA, Horsham.

Sandilands, V., Tolkamp, B.J., Savory, C.J. and Kyriazakis, I. (2006) Behaviour and welfare of broiler breeders fed qualitatively restricted diets during rearing: are there viable alternatives to quantitative restriction? *Applied Animal Behaviour Science* 96, 53–67.

Sandilands, V., Brocklehurst, S., Sparks, N., Baker, L., McGovern, R., Thorp, B. and Pearson, D. (2011) Assessing leg health in chickens using a force plate and gait scoring: how many birds is enough? *Veterinary Record* 168, 77–84.

Sanotra, G.S., Berg, C. and Damkjer Lund, J. (2003) A comparison between leg problems in Danish and Swedish broiler production. *Animal Welfare* 12, 677–683.

Shields, S. and Greger, M. (2013) Animal welfare and food safety aspects of confining broiler chickens to cages. *Animals* 3, 386–400.

Sparrey, J., Sandercock, D.A., Sparks, N.H.C. and Sandilands, V. (2014) Current and novel methods for killing poultry individually on-farm. *World's Poultry Science Journal* 70(4), 737–758.

Stadig, L.M., Rodenburg, T.B., Ampe, B., Reubens, B. and Tuyttens, F.A.M. (2017) Effect of free-range access, shelter type and weather conditions on free-range use and welfare of slow-growing broiler chickens. *Applied Animal Behaviour Science* 192, 15–23.

Svedberg, J. (1996) Report on an Automated Chick Counter. Project report, Swedish Agricultural University, Skara.

Svedberg, J. (1997) Report 1, Chick Separator. Project report, Swedish Agricultural University, Skara.

Svedberg, J. (1998) Report 2, Chick Separator. Project report, Swedish Agricultural University, Skara.

Taylor, P.S., Hemsworth, P.H., Groves, P.J., Gebhardt-Henrich, S.G. and Rault, J.-L. (2017) Ranging behavior of commercial free-range broiler chickens 2: Individual variation. *Animals* 7, 55–64.

Taylor, P.S., Hemsworth, P.H., Groves, P.J., Gebhardt-Henrich, S. and Rault, J.L. (2018) Ranging behavior relates to welfare indicators pre- and post-range access in commercial free-range broilers. *Poultry Science* 97, 1861–1871.

Tong, Q., Demmers, T., Romanini, C., Bergoug, H., Roulston, N., Exadaktylos, V. and McGonnell, I. (2015) Physiological status of broiler chicks at pulling time and the relationship to duration of holding period. *Animal* 9(7), 1181–1187.

Torma, T. and Kovácsné, K.G. (2012) Effects of mechanical impacts on hatchability of broiler breeders. *Journal of Agricultural Science and Technology A* 4, 535–540.

van Emous, R.A., Kwakkel, R., van Krimpen, M. and Hendriks, W. (2015) Effects of different dietary protein levels during rearing and different dietary energy levels during lay on behaviour and feather cover in broiler breeder females. *Applied Animal Behaviour Science* 168, 45–55.

van der Sluis, M., de Klerk, B., Ellen, E.D., de Haas, Y., Hijink, T. and Rodenburg, T.B., (2019) Validation of an ultra-wideband tracking system for recording individual levels of activity in broilers. *Animals: an Open Access Journal from MDPI* 9(8), 580.

Vanderhasselt, R.F., Goethals, K., Buijs, S., Federici, J.F., Sans, E.C.O., Molento, C.F.M., Duchateau, L. and Tuyttens, F.A.M. (2014) Performance of an animal-based test of thirst in commercial broiler chicken farms. *Poultry Science* 93, 1327–1336.

Vasdal, G., Moe, R.O., de Jong, I.C. and, Granquist, E.G. (2018) The relationship between measures of fear of humans and lameness in broiler chicken flocks. *Animal* 12, 334–339.

Velarde, A. and Raj, M. (2016) Gas stunning and killing methods. In: Velarde, A. and Raj, M. (eds) *Animal Welfare at Slaughter.* 5m Publishing, Sheffield, pp. 133–151.

Wallenbeck, A., Wilhelmsson, S., Jönsson, L., Gunnarson, S. and Yngvesson, J. (2016) Behaviour in one fast-growing and one slower-growing hybrid fed a high- or low-protein diet during a 10-week rearing period. *Acta Agriculturae Scandinavica, Section A – Animal Science* 66, 168–176.

Wang, L., Lilburn, M. and Yu, Z. (2016) Intestinal microbiota of broiler chickens as affected by litter management regimens. *Frontiers in Microbiology* 7, Article 593, doi:10.3389/fmicb.2016.00583.

Welfare Quality (2009) *The Welfare Quality Assessment Protocol for Broiler Chickens and Laying Hens.* The Welfare Quality Consortium, Lelystad.

Willemsen, H., Debonne, M,, Swennen, Q., Everaert, N., Careghi, C., Han, H., Bruggeman, V., Tone, K. and Decuypere, E. (2010) Delay in feed access and spread of hatch: importance of early nutrition. *World's Poultry Science Journal* 66, 177–188.

World Health Organization (1948) Official Records of the World Health Organization, no. 2. WHO, Geneva.

Yang, Y., Pan, C., Zhong, R. and Pan, J. (2018) Artificial light and biological responses of broiler chickens: dose-response. *Journal of Animal Science* 96, 98–107.

Index